A
CLINICIAN'S
DICTIONARY
OF PATHOGENIC
MICROORGANISMS

A
CLINICIAN'S
DICTIONARY
OF PATHOGENIC
MICROORGANISMS

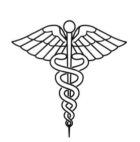

James H. Jorgensen

Professor of Pathology, Medicine, Microbiology, and
    Clinical Laboratory Sciences
The University of Texas Health Science Center
Director, Microbiology Laboratory
University Hospital
San Antonio, Texas

AND

Michael A. Pfaller

Professor of Pathology and Epidemiology
Director, Molecular Epidemiology and Fungus Testing Laboratory
The University of Iowa College of Medicine and
    College of Public Health
Iowa City, Iowa

ASM PRESS

WASHINGTON, D.C.

Address editorial correspondence to ASM Press, 1752 N St., N.W., Washington, DC 20036-2904, USA

Send orders to ASM Press, P.O. Box 605, Herndon, VA 20172, USA
Phone: 800-546-2416; 703-661-1593
Fax: 703-661-1501
E-mail: books@asmusa.org
Online : www.asmpress.org

Library of Congress Cataloging-in-Publication Data

Jorgensen, James H.
   A clinician's dictionary of pathogenic microorganisms / James H. Jorgensen and Michael A. Pfaller.
        p. ; cm.
Includes bibliographical references and index.
   ISBN 1-55581-280-5
   1. Pathogenic microorganisms–Dictionaries. 2. Microbiology–Classification–Dictionaries.
   [DNLM: 1. Bacteria–Dictionary–English. 2. Fungi–Dictionary–English. 3. Parasites–Dictionary–English. 4. Viruses–Dictionary–English. QW 13 J82c 2003] I. Pfaller, Michael A. II. Title.
   QR81.J67 2003
   616.9′041′03–dc22

                                        2003015175

10 9 8 7 6 5 4 3 2 1

Contents

Preface

This booklet represents an attempt to provide clinicians with a convenient means of understanding the taxonomic designations of the various bacteria, mycobacteria, fungi, parasites, and viruses that may be recovered from their patients. The taxonomy (the names of the microorganisms) continues to be updated and changed with alarming frequency. Much of this is based on our expanding knowledge of the ability of certain "newer" organism groups to cause disease, e.g., *Helicobacter* species, *Bartonella* species, *Rhodococcus* species, *Ehrlichia*, *Cyclospora*, and hepatitis viruses. In addition, application of the powerful new tools of molecular biology to groups of organisms such as the family *Enterobacteriaceae* has led to reclassification of older members of the family and to description of newly recognized species based on the homology of their DNA. This booklet catalogues the current state of microbial taxonomy as of mid-2003.

Considerable effort has gone into making this catalogue of pathogenic microorganisms as complete as possible. It should be regarded as a "quick reference," however, and, thus, a starting place to gain an understanding of the significance of the recovery of various microbes from human clinical specimens. An attempt has been made to include all of the common pathogens, and several less frequent ones. However, it is not an exhaustive listing of arcane microorganisms. The reference lists included in the booklet present a selection of the most contemporary sources (mainly books, reviews, and the most clinically relevant journal articles) that the reader may pursue for a more in-depth discussion of the various organisms and diseases.

We sincerely hope that this dictionary will help increase the understanding of microbial pathogens by practicing clinicians, house officers, students, epidemiologists, infection control practitioners, and other allied health professionals. It is to their need for concise, practical information that we have directed this effort.

JAMES H. JORGENSEN, Ph.D.
MICHAEL A. PFALLER, M.D.
May 2003

Bacteria

Abiotrophia. A relatively new genus composed of gram-positive cocci that were formerly referred to as "nutritionally deficient" or "satelliting" streptococci. They were originally considered to be nutritionally defective members of the viridans group of streptococci. However, a new genus and species has been recognized, i.e., *Abiotrophia defectiva* (48). This organism is most notable as a cause of bacteremia or endocarditis, and it may be somewhat more difficult to eradicate with antibiotics than streptococci. See also the closely related genus, *Granulacatella.*

Achromobacter. A genus of aerobic gram-negative bacilli that do not ferment glucose and, thus, do not belong to the family *Enterobacteriaceae.* Several members of the genus have been classified intermittently as *Achromobacter* or *Alcaligenes* species. They are probably part of the normal lower gastrointestinal flora. *Achromobacter* species are a cause of occasional nosocomial infections, and are isolated primarily from urine, wounds, sputum, and occasionally blood. Resistance to antibiotics, including aminoglycosides, is frequently demonstrated. There are three species or subspecies designations of the most important species.

A. piechaudii. A species that has been recovered from occasional cases of bacteremia, respiratory specimens, and the environment.

A. xylosoxidans subsp. *xylosoxidans.* A relatively frequent isolate from nosocomial infections, in particular, in patients with pneumonia or bacteremia. It is also an occasional cause of pulmonary infection in patients with cystic fibrosis or adults with preexisting lung disease (26).

A. xylosoxidans subsp. *denitrificans.* Formerly classified as *Alcaligenes denitrificans* and an occasional cause of various nosocomial infections.

Acinetobacter. Genus of aerobic gram-negative coccobacilli that do not ferment glucose and do not belong to the family *Enterobacteriaceae. Acinetobacter* species are the second most frequently isolated group of nonfermentative gram-negative bacilli. They are widely distributed in nature in water, soil, and sewage, and in the hospital environment. They can be recovered as a colonizer from most areas of the human body, including the skin, and may cause opportunistic infections, especially in debilitated individuals. Because of similar size and shape of cells, *Acinetobacter* species may be mistaken for *Neisseria* species in smears of spinal fluid or pus.

A. baumannii. Part of the *A. calcoaceticus-A. baumannii* complex. (Because of practical difficulties in identifying this organism, it may be reported as *A. calcoaceticus* var. *anitratus* or simply as *A. anitratus*.) It is an opportunistic pathogen associated with nosocomial pneumonia, urinary tract infections, wound infections, and septicemia, and may be found to contaminate equipment for inhalation therapy and renal dialysis (7). *A. baumannii* may be harbored in the gastrointestinal tract of hospitalized patients. It is resistant to antimicrobial agents more often than *A. calcoaceticus* var. *lwoffii*.

A. calcoaceticus var. *lwoffii* (or simply A. *lwoffii*). Can be part of the normal flora of the skin and gastrointestinal tract, and is found in nature and the hospital environment. It is isolated less frequently from nosocomial infections than *A. baumannii* and, in general, is more susceptible to antimicrobial agents. There are several other newly described species of *Acinetobacter* that are of uncertain clinical significance.

Actinobacillus. Genus of fastidious gram-negative coccobacilli previously thought to be associated with actinomycosis. They are colonizers of the respiratory and genitourinary tracts of animals and humans, and they can cause septicemic infections in humans and a variety of animals.

   A. actinomycetemcomitans. Associated historically with actinomycosis, but only rarely found in actinomycotic soft tissue lesions with *Actinomyces* spp. It is part of the normal flora of the human mouth, but also a cause of periodontitis. It has been isolated most often from humans with bacterial endocarditis and from abscesses of the brain and soft tissues. It is morphologically and biochemically related to *Haemophilus*, and it represents the "A" in the HACEK group acronym (19).

   A. equuli and ***A. suis.*** Part of the normal mouth flora of horses and swine, but also a cause of septicemia, arthritis, and nephritis in foals and pigs. They are a rare cause of wound infections in humans.

A. hominis and *A. ureae.* Opportunistic pathogens of the respiratory tract of debilitated people and are occasionally associated with septicemia in humans.

A. lignieresii. The causative organism of actino-bacillosis or "wooden tongue" in cattle and sheep, and has produced a few human infections, including abscesses, septicemia, and endocarditis. It is part of the normal flora of the mouths of cattle and sheep, but it is most commonly a cause of wound infections in humans.

Actinomadura. Genus of aerobic actinomycete that is distributed worldwide, but is most common in tropical and subtropical areas. Like *Actinomyces*, *Actinomadura* is a cause of mycetomas of the extremities following injury or exposure to soil or water.

Actinomyces. Genus of anaerobic gram-positive bacilli with structural branching resembling that of a fungus. *Actinomyces* is the etiologic agent of actino-mycosis in humans and animals (70). Among animals, the infection is most common in cattle (lumpy jaw).

A. israelii. Part of the normal flora of the human mouth and probably of the gastrointestinal tract and vagina. It produces a chronic disease with abscesses and draining sinuses, most frequently in the skin and subcutaneous tissues of the head and neck. Infection may follow tooth extraction or injury in the mouth. *A. israelii* can cause primary lesions in the lungs, with abscesses and empyema, or in the abdomen. Serious pelvic infections due to *Actinomyces* have occurred in women fitted with intrauterine devices (IUDs) for contraception (33). Wound drainage often contains small yellow or brown "sulfur granules."

***A. naeslundii*, *A. odontolyticus*, *A. viscosus*, *A. meyeri*, *A. turicensis*, *A. radingae*, and *A. neuii*.** Species also inhabiting the human mouth and intestine. They are less common causes of subcutaneous or pulmonary infections in humans than *A. israelii*.

Aerococcus. A genus of gram-positive cocci that may be found in soil or water or occasionally on human skin. It closely resembles the enterococci. There are two principal species, *A. viridans* and *A. urinae*. *Aerococcus* may cause urinary tract infections, bacteremia, and endocarditis.

Aeromonas. Genus of aerobic gram-negative bacilli normally found in fresh water, brackish water, soil, and sewage. Cold-blooded animals and humans can become infected.

A. caviae. One of the most common causes of usually mild, self-limited gastrointestinal infections, particularly in children, in addition to diarrhea, abdominal pain, vomiting, and fever.

A. hydrophila. Occurs naturally in fresh water and soil. It is carried in the gastrointestinal tract of some healthy individuals, and it can cause acute diarrheal disease, mostly in the summer months. Hemolytic-uremic syndrome may occasionally follow *Aeromonas* diarrhea. Most common are wound infections and cellulitis following trauma associated with water or soil contamination. In immunosuppressed individuals, wound infections can be severe, resembling clostridial myonecrosis. *Aeromonas* septicemia may develop in patients with chronic hepatic disease and is associated with a high mortality rate. Other infections include ocular, lower respiratory tract, and urinary tract infections, as well as osteomyelitis, septic arthritis, otitis, endocarditis, and meningitis (3).

A. shigelloides. See *Plesiomonas shigelloides*.

A. veronii biovar **sobria** (or simply **A. sobria**). Produces a severe cholera-like disease with abdominal pain, profuse diarrhea, nausea, and fever. This species has also caused wound infections associated with the use of medicinal leeches.

Afipia. *Afipia* presently includes only one species, *A. felis*, a fastidious gram-negative rod that was initially described as the cause of cat scratch disease (CSD). More recent data suggest that *Bartonella henselae* is the causative agent of most cases of CSD.

Agrobacterium. Genus of gram-negative, non-glucose-fermentative bacilli that are primarily plant pathogens that occasionally infect humans through contact with soil or water. *A. radiobacter* has been recovered from peritoneal dialysate, ascites fluid, catheter tips, urine, and blood. Isolates are generally not highly antibiotic resistant (28).

Alcaligenes. Genus of gram-negative, non-glucose-fermentative bacilli that are normally found in water and soil. They may be found in moist areas within the hospital environment, such as respirators and dialyzers, and are occasionally isolated from persons with urinary tract infections, pneumonia, or septicemia. *Alcaligenes* and *Achromobacter* are closely related genera.

   A. faecalis. The most common species of *Alcaligenes*. It occasionally causes urinary tract infections and, in debilitated individuals, pneumonia and septicemia.

A. denitrificans. Now classified as *Achromobacter xylosoxidans* subsp. *denitrificans.*

A. odorans. Now included in *A. faecalis.* It is notable for producing an odor of freshly sliced green apples.

Alkalescens-Dispar group. Gram-negative rods intermediate in evolution between *Escherichia coli* and *Shigella.* They are most often included as a serotype of *E. coli.*

Alloiococcus. A recently described genus of slow-growing, aerobic gram-positive cocci that resemble staphylococci. The only species, *A. otitidis*, has been implicated as a cause of chronic otitis media in children (29).

Anaplasma. Anaplasma phagocytophylum is an obligate intracellular bacterium that previously was considered a species of *Ehrlichia.* It is the causative organism of the tick-borne disease, human granulo-cytic ehrlichiosis (HE). Similar to human monocyto-tropic ehrlichiosis, it is characterized by high fever, myalgia, malaise, headache, but with a rash in only about 10% of patients. Complications can include adult respiratory distress syndrome and septic shock (4).

Arachnia propionica. Species of gram-positive anaerobic or microaerophilic rods now classified as *Propionibacterium propionica*.

Arcanobacterium. A genus of aerobic gram-positive rods that are closely related to both *Corynebacterium* and *Actinomyces*.

> ***A. bernardiae.*** Close resemblance to *A. pyogenes*.

> ***A. haemolyticum.*** A cause of pharyngitis in older children and adolescents, and of wound infections, osteomyelitis, and septicemia in various age groups. Its in vitro growth characteristics closely mimic those of β-hemolytic streptococci (59).

> ***A. pyogenes.*** A cause of abscesses and bacteremia in humans and animals.

Arcobacter. A genus of curved gram-negative bacilli closely related to (and formerly classified as) *Campylobacter*. *A. butzleri* and *A. cryaerophilus* may cause diarrhea and bacteremia in some immunosuppressed patients.

Arthrobacter. A genus of uncommon coryneform gram-positive bacteria that are normal skin inhabitants, and occasionally cause foreign body infections and bacteremia.

Arizona. Taxonomists continue to debate whether *Arizona hinshawii* or *Salmonella arizonae* is a more correct name for this close relative of *Salmonella*. This genus may cause gastroenteritis or bacteremia in a manner similar to that of *Salmonella*. Cases are often associated with the care and handling of turtles or snakes.

Bacillus. Genus of large, gram-positive, spore-forming aerobic or facultative rods, most species of which are saprophytes found in soil and water. It represents a common laboratory contaminant but is also an occasional pathogen of humans and animals. Many species have been described, but the following species are of greatest significance.

B. anthracis. A large rod with subterminal spores that causes anthrax in cattle, sheep, and horses. Humans are occasionally infected in nature by spores that enter through injured skin or mucous membranes and, less frequently, through inhalation. *B. anthracis* produces skin infection (malignant pustule), septicemia, pneumonia (wool-sorters' disease), enteritis (not reported in the United States), and meningitis. Most recently, it has been considered an important agent of biological terrorism and warfare.

B. Calmette-Guérin (BCG). Not a *Bacillus* sp. See *Mycobacterium bovis*.

B. cereus. A species with subterminal spores. It is widely distributed in nature in dust and soil, on plants, and in milk. It is one cause of toxin-mediated "food poisoning" and has caused traumatic wound infections, corneal infections, catheter infections, pneumonia, endocarditis, and osteomyelitis (25). *B. cereus* is perhaps the most commonly isolated *Bacillus* species. It usually produces a potent β-lactamase, making it resistant to many penicillins and cephalosporins.

B. megaterium. Has subterminal spores. It is widely distributed in nature in soil, water, dust, and decomposing matter. It is rarely isolated from infectious processes.

B. subtilis. Has subterminal spores. It is often present in soil, decomposing matter, dust, and air, and is a frequent laboratory contaminant. It may secondarily contaminate wounds, and it has rarely caused septicemia, pneumonitis, meningitis, and endocarditis.

Other *Bacillus* spp. that may cause occasional infections in humans, such as wound or corneal infections, bacteremia, or meningitis include

B. circulans, B. coagulans, B. pumilis, B. sphaer-icus, B. thiuringiensis, and *B. brevis.*

Bacteroides. The most important genus of anaerobic gram-negative rods, usually found as a large part of normal fecal flora. *Bacteroides* is also found in the lower genitourinary tract and less commonly in the oropharynx. Along with species of *Clostridium, Bacteroides* spp. are the most frequently isolated and most clinically significant anaerobic bacteria. The taxonomy of the gram-negative anaerobic bacteria has undergone almost constant revision during the past few years, causing great confusion for both microbiologists and clinicians.

B. corrodens. Now known as *Bacteroides ureolyticus.*

B. fragilis group. The group that usually consti-tutes about 95% of normal fecal flora and is also part of the normal flora of the genital tract. When associated with disease, it is often part of a mixture of anaerobes and aerobes. The *B. fragilis* group has been isolated from various intra-abdominal infec-tions, appendicitis, peritonitis, rectal abscesses, breast abscesses, pilonidal cysts, postsurgical wound infections, endometritis, puerperal sepsis, salpingitis, septicemia (with metastatic abscesses to brain, lungs, etc.), and pneumonia with empyema

(32). Members of this group are more resistant to antimicrobial agents than other anaerobes, in large part, due to production of a potent β-lactamase affecting penicillin and several members of the cephalosporin class. Individual species of the *B. fragilis* group include: *B. caccae, B. distasonis, B. eggerthii, B. fragilis, B. merdae, B. ovatus, B. stercoris, B. thetaiotaomicron, B. uniformis,* and *B. vulgatus.*

B. fragilis. The most virulent species of the *B. fragilis* group because of its polysaccharide capsule, ability to produce destructive extracellular enzymes (including an enterotoxin), and potent β-lactamases (32).

B. gracilis. Now included in the genera *Campylobacter* or *Sutterella.*

B. thetaiotaomicron. The second most important and often most antibiotic-resistant species of the *B. fragilis* group.

Other *Bacteroides* species. There are several other members of the genus that are involved less often in infections in humans, but may occasionally be isolated. These include primarily *B. capillosis* and *B. coagulans.*

Balneatrix. An aerobic gram-negative rod that is a very rare cause of hot-spring-spa–associated infections, including respiratory and bloodstream infections.

Bartonella. Genus of small, highly fastidious gram-negative bacilli that cause bacteremia, endocarditis, bacillary angiomatosis, and in particular, cat scratch disease. There are now 16 species, but the two species described below are the most common and clinically significant.

> ***B. henselae.*** The best-documented etiologic agent of cat scratch disease, bacillary angiomatosis, peliosis, and occasionally, it is a cause of endocarditis. It causes a nonfatal bacteremia in young cats, and appears to be spread from cat to cat and to humans by fleas. Formerly known as *Rochalimaea henselae*, it has now been renamed as *B. henselae* (22, 74). Occasional cases of cat scratch disease may be caused by another species, *B. clarridgeiae*.

> ***B. quintana.*** Causes a febrile, bacteremic infection called trench fever. It is transmitted by lice, and it is associated with poor hygiene and living conditions.

Bedsonia. Old name for *Chlamydia*.

Bergeyella. A new genus of aerobic gram-negative rods that was recently classified as *Weeksella zoohelcum*. Now, reclassified as *B. zoohelcum*, it is associated with wound infections from dog or cat bites. Some patients have progressed to bacteremia and meningitis.

Bifidobacterium. Genus of gram-positive, non-spore-forming, anaerobic rods. It may be isolated from the mucous membranes and the intestine of humans. Occasionally, the organism is associated with abscesses and pulmonary disease and may be confused with *Actinomyces* because of the bifurcated appearance of some cells that may resemble the branching morphology of *Actinomyces*. The most common species appears to be *B. dentium*.

Bilophila. Presently, there is only one species, *B. wadsworthia*, an anaerobic gram-negative rod that has been associated most often with gangrenous or perforated appendicitis or other intra-abdominal infections (32). It has also been a cause of bacteremia and focal abscesses. Because it is fastidious and slow growing in vitro, *B. wadsworthia* may not be isolated as frequently as other gram-negative anaerobes, e.g., *Bacteroides* spp.

Bordetella. Genus of small, aerobic gram-negative coccobacilli, or rods, similar in appearance to

Brucella and *Haemophilus*. There are now seven recognized species, including those described below.

B. bronchiseptica. May be part of the normal flora in the respiratory tract of humans, dogs, rabbits, swine, horses, and other animals. It causes kennel cough in dogs and atrophic rhinitis in swine. It can cause chronic pneumonitis or wound infections in humans, especially those who are immuno-suppressed.

B. hinzii. Colonizes the respiratory tract of poultry. It has rarely been isolated from the secretions of the respiratory tract in humans.

B. holmesii. A rare cause of respiratory diseases, including a pertussis-like syndrome.

B. parapertussis. Produces a disease similar to, but milder than, whooping cough. It is found in both humans and lambs.

B. pertussis. The etiologic agent of the toxin-mediated disease pertussis (whooping cough) and is occasionally isolated from patients with interstitial pneumonia. It may be isolated from the nasophar-yngeal secretions of infected patients, but only by means of specialized culture media that satisfy the organism's fastidious growth requirements.

Borrelia. Genus of spirochetal gram-negative micro-organisms of the family *Spirochaetaceae.* All *Borrelia* are arthropod-borne, including those that cause relapsing fever and Lyme disease. Most species cannot be cultured in vitro with standard culture media.

B. burgdorferi (and several proposed subspecies). The causative agent of Lyme disease or borreliosis, a multisystem complex of symptoms, starting with erythema migrans, progressing to hematogenous dissemination in some patients, and later including meningitis and facial nerve palsy. Lyme arthritis can occur months to years after the initial infection (5, 15). It is transmitted primarily by Ixodid ticks. *B. burgdorferi* was not proven as the agent of Lyme disease until it was isolated in culture in 1981 (80). Genetic hybridization studies have led recently to the naming of several subspecies or variants, including *B. garinii* and *B. afzelii.* Accurate diagnosis is complex, and relies on a series of immunologic and molecular tests.

B. recurrentis. The most common cause of louse-borne relapsing fever in humans. Other relapsing fever borreliae are transmitted by soft ticks. Infections are characterized by high fever, shaking chills, headache, myalgia, malaise, and nausea. Fever attacks often last for 3 to 7 days, separated by several days or even weeks. Louse-borne disease is generally more severe than tick-borne relapsing fever.

Branhamella. See *Moraxella catarrhalis.*

Brevibacterium. Coryneform gram-positive bacilli best known as part of the normal skin flora. Perhaps the most interesting aspect of the genus is that most strains give off a distinctive cheese-like odor when grown in culture.

Brevundimonas. *Brevundimonas vesicularis* is a non-glucose-fermentative, gram-negative rod that used to be classified as a *Pseudomonas* species. It is an occasional cause of nosocomial infections, including bacteremia.

Brucella. Genus of fastidious, extremely small gram-negative coccobacilli that are intracellular parasites capable of infecting many animal hosts, including humans. Brucellosis is a zoonotic infection also known as undulant fever or Malta fever. Each species has a preferred host (*B. melitensis*, sheep and goats; *B. suis*, swine; *B. abortus*, cattle; *B. canis*, dogs), but all can infect several animal species including humans. Humans can be infected through ingestion of contaminated milk products including cheese, through inhalation of droplets onto mucous membranes, or through skin contact with infected products or tissues.

Brucella species are most frequently isolated from patients' blood during febrile periods, and may also be recovered from bone marrow, exudates, lymph nodes, urine, peritoneal fluid, cerebrospinal fluid, and the placenta. They can produce granulomas or abscesses in tissues of the reticuloendothelial system, osteomyelitis, meningitis, cholecystitis, pneumonitis, endocarditis, and skin, mouth, and eye lesions. In addition, *Brucella* species have been considered as possible agents of bioterrorism.

Burkholderia. A genus of non-glucose-fermentative, gram-negative bacilli that most recently were part of the genus *Pseudomonas*. They were reclassified on the basis of DNA-relatedness studies.

> **B. cepacia.** The most commonly isolated member of the genus, and is a well-recognized nosocomial pathogen that causes urinary tract infections, pneumonia, catheter infections, peritonitis, bacteremia, and meningitis. It is often associated with contaminated hospital equipment or solutions (including disinfectants and nebulizer solutions). In addition, *B. cepacia* has been recognized as an important pathogen in patients with cystic fibrosis and chronic granulomatous disease (57).

> **B. gladioli.** Causes infections very similar to those caused by *B. cepacia*.

B. mallei. The causative organism of glanders (a disease of horses), which may very rarely be transmitted to humans by direct contact or inhalation.

B. pseudomallei. The etiologic agent of melioidosis, which may present as a chronic lung disease or as overwhelming septicemia, or it may be asymptomatic for years (54). Abscesses may develop in the viscera, bone, or skin following contact with contaminated soil or water, or may be contracted by aerosolization of water. The organism can cause disease that resembles tuberculosis, including the possibility of latent infections due to chronic underlying conditions (e.g., liver disease, diabetes). The usual habitat of *B. pseudomallei* is surface waters of Southeast Asia and Northern Australia, moist soil, and the surfaces of fruits and vegetables in those areas. It is rarely the cause of infection in the United States, but is a possible agent of bioterrorism.

Buttiauxella. A recently described, but infrequently encountered member of the family *Enterobacteriaceae*.

***Calymmatobacterium granulomatis* (formerly *Donovania granulomatis*).** Species of large gramnegative, pleomorphic coccobacilli with prominent polar granules ("safety pin" appearance). *C. granulomatis* produces the tropical venereal disease granuloma inguinale, with ulcerating granulomatous lesions in skin and subcutaneous tissues, and with possible secondary involvement of bones and joints. In general, diagnosis is made by histologic examination for Donovan bodies. At present, it is not culturable.

Campylobacter. Genus of microaerophilic or anaerobic gram-negative, curved rods that may occur in short chains resembling spirals or gull wings; originally placed in the genus *Vibrio*. The most important species are listed below.

C. coli. Causes disease in humans that is indistinguishable from that caused by *C. jejuni*.

C. fetus (formerly *Vibrio fetus; C. intestinalis*). First described in cattle and sheep, in which it caused a venereal disease that resulted in abortions and decreased conception rates. Now, it is known also to produce brucellosis-like human infections, including septicemia, meningitis, and endocarditis. Those factors predisposing to infection, such as neoplasm or cirrhosis, often are present.

C. jejuni. A common inhabitant of the gastrointestinal tract of many warm-blooded animals, including poultry, cattle, sheep, horses, dogs, cats, etc. Now, it is recognized as the most common bacterial agent of acute gastroenteritis in humans in the United States; it is acquired through ingestion of unpasteurized milk or improperly cooked poultry or meat, or by direct contact with infected animals or humans (10, 96). It is also recognized as an antecedent cause of Guillain-Barré syndrome due to some cross-reacting antibodies. Reactive arthritis and Reiter's syndrome may occur in days to weeks after a *Campylobacter* infection. Although special media and conditions are required for isolation of *C. jejuni,* it should be routinely sought in the diagnosis of infectious diarrhea. Occasional extraintestinal infections occur, including bacteremia, meningitis, septic arthritis, and various abscesses.

C. lari. A thermophilic *Campylobacter* species normally found in avian species, especially seagulls. It may cause gastrointestinal or systemic infections in humans.

C. pylori. See *Helicobacter pylori.*

C. upsaliensis. A less frequent cause of diarrhea and bacteremia.

C. gracilis, C. curvus, and *C. rectus.* Obligate anaerobes that were previously classified as *Bacteroides* species. They have been associated mainly with oral or periodontal infections, or other infections of the head and neck.

Several other species of *Campylobacter* have been described, often as part of the intestinal or oral flora of humans and various animals. However, their disease-producing abilities have not been firmly established at this time.

Capnocytophaga. Gram-negative facultative or anaerobic, fastidious gram-negative bacilli that often appear as long pointed or spindle-shaped cells. Some species demonstrate an unusual "gliding motility." Several species are associated with periodontal disease, but may cause systemic infections in debilitated individuals, while some species are associated with animal contact. The most common species are listed below.

C. canimorsus (formerly CDC group DF-2). Causes infections in wounds from animal bites (particularly dog bites) that can lead to severe, fulminant septicemia, possibly resulting in death in splenectomized patients or those with preexisting liver disease (alcoholics) (14, 66). *C. cynodegmi* is also a cause of localized infections due to dog bites, usually without severe, systemic infection.

C. gingivalis, C. granulosa, C. haemolytica, C. ochracea, and C. sputagena are members of the human oral flora C. gingivalis, C. ochracea, and C. sputagena are associated with periodontitis.

Cardiobacterium hominis. Species of fastidious gram-negative, pleomorphic bacilli that may be part of the normal flora of the nasopharynx and, less commonly, of the vagina and cervix of some individuals. C. hominis has caused endocarditis, and rarely meningitis. It is the "C" of the HACEK group of organisms (19).

CDC "groups." Prior to extensive DNA homology and detailed phenotypic studies, newly recognized or uncommon organisms may be listed by a CDC "number" (e.g., IIc, IIe, IIg, IVc, IVe, etc.). Many times these are non-glucose-fermentative, gram-negative bacilli associated with moist environments. As more strains, and hence more data, are collected, these isolates eventually receive genus and species designations.

Cedecea. Recently described genus of the family *Enterobacteriaceae.* Only rarely encountered in

clinical specimens, such as urine. Species include
C. davisae and *C. lapagei.*

Cellulomonas. A genus of gram-positive, non-spore-forming aerobic rods related to the corynebacteria.
C. hominis has been an infrequent cause of
bacteremia.

Chlamydiae (formerly Bedsoniae). Small, obligate,
intracellular, gram-negative bacteria of the psittaco-sis-lymphogranuloma venereum (LGV)-trachoma-inclusion conjunctivitis intracytoplasmic organism
group. *Chlamydia* species were once considered
viruses because of their small size. They have a unique
growth cycle that distinguishes them from all other
microorganisms. Their life cycle consists of metabol-ically inactive, infectious elements (elementary bodies)
and metabolically active, but noninfectious reticulate
bodies. The former *Chlamydia pneumoniae* has been
transferred to the genus *Chlamydophila.*

  C. psittaci is the cause of psittacosis (ornithosis), a
  disease of birds and other animals that may be
  transferred to humans by aerosols from contami-nated feces. Psittacosis results in varying manifes-tations, ranging from inapparent infections to
  severe pneumonia, with septicemia, endocarditis,
  or meningitis.

C. trachomatis (TRIC agent, LGV *Chlamydia*) is the most common bacterial cause of sexually transmitted disease in developed countries (more common than gonorrhea). *C. trachomatis* serovars D through K cause nongonococcal urethritis and epididymitis in men; proctitis, conjunctivitis, and Reiter's syndrome; and cervicitis, endometritis, and salpingitis in women. The salpingitis is a major cause of infertility or tubal pregnancy. Infants may contract eye infections or pneumonia during passage through the birth canal of an infected mother. Serovars A, B, Ba, and C are associated with endemic trachoma or inclusion conjunctivitis (inclusion blenorrhea). Trachoma typically involves the upper eyelid and may lead to scar formation over the cornea and eventually to blindness. Serovars L1, L2, and L3 cause the important sexually transmitted diseases, lymphogranuloma venereum (LGV) or lymphopathia venereum.

Chlamydophila. *Chlamydophila pneumoniae* is a small, obligate, intracellular, gram-negative bacterium formerly classified as *Chlamydia pneumoniae*, and before that known as the TWAR agent. It causes a variety of respiratory symptoms from pharyngitis, bronchitis, and exacerbations of asthma, to community-acquired pneumonia. Together with *Mycoplasma pneumoniae*, *C. pneumoniae* is thought to be a very common cause of lower respiratory tract infections in all age groups. Also of note are several publications that suggest a possible role for *C. pneumoniae* infection in the development of atherosclerosis, coronary heart disease, stroke, Alzheimer's disease, and multiple sclerosis (77, 95).

Chromobacterium violaceum. Species of facultative, glucose-fermenting, nonenteric, gram-negative rods that form violet colony pigments. It most often is saprophytic and is found in soil and water. *C. violaceum* has produced skin lesions, abscesses, urinary tract infections, septicemia, and meningitis in humans.

Chryseobacterium. A newly described genus, formed primarily from the genus *Flavobacterium*. The natural habitat of these aerobic gram-negative, yellow-pigmented bacteria is soil or water. They are occasional causes of nosocomial infections due to their presence in tap water.

   C. indologenes. A rare cause of bacteremia associated with catheter or intravenous fluid contamination.

   C. meningosepticum. Causes bacteremia and meningitis in premature neonates, and occasionally pneumonia and bacteremia in adults (11).

Chryseomonas. Primarily *C. luteola* (formerly *Pseu-domonas luteola*), a gram-negative rod that is a rare cause of nosocomial infection.

Citrobacter. Genus of gram-negative rods of the family *Enterobacteriaceae* somewhat resembling *Salmonella*. It has been isolated from water and sewage and from the feces of healthy persons, and it has been associated with many different types of extraintestinal infections (often hospital-acquired) (24).

C. amalonaticus. One of the most recently described species of *Citrobacter*. It has caused urinary tract infections and bacteremia.

C. diversus. Now known as *C. koseri*.

C. freundii. The most commonly encountered and most antibiotic-resistant species. It is a cause of urinary tract and wound infections, pneumonia, bacteremia, and meningitis.

C. koseri. The newer designation for *C. diversus*. *C. koseri* may be mistaken at times for *E. coli* because of some common biochemical characteristics. It has caused urinary tract infections, wound infections, pneumonia, and bacteremia. It is known in particular as a cause of meningitis in children less than 2 months of age (56).

There are several other *Citrobacter* species that are rarely associated with infections in humans.

Clostridium. Genus of anaerobic, large, gram-positive, spore-forming rods. Most *Clostridium* species are soil, water, and sewage saprophytes. Some *Clostridium* species form part of the normal intestinal flora of humans and many animals, and many decompose protein and/or produce toxins. Those species associated with human disease can be divided into five main disease groups.

1. Gas gangrene or wound infections, including myonecrosis (in order of decreasing frequency). *C. perfringens, C. septicum, C. histolyticum, C. bifermentans,* and *C. novyi,* and, less often, *C. sordellii, C. fallax, C. sporogenes,* and *C. tertium.* Bacteremia without gas gangrene can occur following bowel surgery or necrosis.

2. Botulism. *C. botulinum* includes types A through G, based on immunologic specificity of the unique neuroparalytic toxin [now called botulism neurotoxin (BoNT)], that is one of the most highly toxic substances known. BoNT types A, B, and E are most frequently associated with human disease. Four types of clinical botulism are recognized. First, it classically occurs when preformed toxin in foods is ingested. The organism is normally found in soil and, occasionally, in animal feces. Vegetables and fruits are often contaminated with spores. Botulism toxin is heat labile. Second, wound botulism may occur by local toxin production in an infected wound. Third, infant botulism is now the most frequently encountered form of the disease; apparently, it results from toxin production within the bowel of affected infants (possibly following ingestion of honey contaminated with C. *botulinum* spores). The fourth type is in vivo toxin production in the bowel of adults and children. In addition, three other related clostridial species have been shown to have the capability of producing BoNT. C. *butyricum* can produce BoNT type E, C. *baratii* can produce type F, and C. *argentinense* can produce type G toxin. Furthermore, there is now a fifth form of botulism, inhalational, that can occur with aerosolization of the purified toxin as a bioterrorism weapon.

3. Tetanus. C. *tetani* has a large terminal spore that produces a drumstick or tennis racket appearance. The organism is found in soil and animal feces. Initial infection often occurs from a puncture wound contaminated with soil. Tetanus results from a toxemia, with the neurotoxin (tetanospasmin) acting on nerve tissue of the spinal cord and peripheral nerves (lockjaw, risus sardonicus).

4. *C. difficile.* The cause of many cases of antibiotic-associated diarrhea (AAD) and antibiotic-induced pseudomembranous enterocolitis (45). *C. difficile*-associated disease (CDAD) appears to be the first step that occurs when natural bowel colonization with *C. difficile* is amplified in the presence of antibiotic therapy, principally in hospitalized patients. Local production of at least two different toxins (toxins A and B) leads to diarrhea and local inflammation of the bowel. CDAD may be diagnosed by culture or by detection of its specific toxins in feces.

5. *C. perfringens.* In addition to causing gas gangrene and other suppurative conditions, is perhaps the most common cause of "food poisoning" due to production of an enterotoxin in certain foods, especially meats, that results in crampy abdominal pain and diarrhea (75). Other gastrointestinal maladies include antibiotic-induced diarrhea and enteritis necrotans. The latter condition (also called "pig-bel") is due to β-toxin-producing strains that cause a life-threatening necrosis of the small bowel. It is a condition that is largely limited to developing countries, but has been reported in the United States. Last, it has been speculated that *C. perfringens* may have a role in necrotizing enterocolitis in neonates.

6. *C. septicum.* Bacteremia appears to result from escape of the organism from the bowel into the bloodstream due to bowel damage from various malignancies, especially leukemia, lymphoma, and carcinoma of the colon (50). Such patients may be neutropenic, and can suffer rapid severe disease with a high mortality rate.

Coliforms. General term applied to some species of the family *Enterobacteriaceae,* usually *Escherichia coli* and *Citrobacter, Enterobacter,* and *Klebsiella* species.

Comamonas. Gram-negative, non-glucose-fermentative rod previously classified as a species of *Pseudomonas.* The primary species is *C. testosteroni.* It is commonly found in the environment, i.e., soil and water.

Corynebacterium. Genus of aerobic, gram-positive, club-shaped rods, sometimes with irregular granules, often appearing in palisade arrangements (Chinese letters, picket fence). Widely distributed in nature in soil, plants, and animals. Many species are part of the normal flora of the skin, respiratory tract, and mucous membranes, but several species are pathogenic for humans and animals.

C. acnes. See *Propionibacterium acnes.*

C. amycolatum. One of the most commonly isolated species, perhaps because it is a member of the normal skin flora. It is often multiply antibiotic resistant.

C. diphtheriae (**Klebs-Loeffler bacillus**). The causative agent of diphtheria; its potent exotoxin produces many pathologic effects, primarily on the heart and peripheral nerves. Most cases result from infection of the upper respiratory tract, but cutaneous infections also occur in tropical climates. It may exist in the respiratory tract, skin, or wounds of healthy carriers.

C. equi. See *Rhodococcus.*

C. jeikeium (**formerly Group JK**). A relatively common cause of catheter infections, wound infections, bacteremia, and endocarditis. It is a very antibiotic resistant species, often infecting debilitated patients (40).

C. pseudodiphtheriticum (**formerly *C. hofmanii***). May be a part of the normal throat flora. It is very rarely reported as a cause of pneumonia.

C. pseudotuberculosis. Has been isolated from chronic purulent lesions in horses, sheep, and goats and has occasionally infected humans. It is a close relative of *C. diphtheriae*, and some strains can produce diphtheria toxin.

C. striatum. Part of the normal skin flora. It may cause nosocomial infections such as those involving intravenous catheters.

C. ulcerans. Has been isolated from exudative pharyngitis causing a diphtheria-like disease.

C. urealyticum. A cause of urinary tract and wound infections, bacteremia, and endocarditis. It is often quite antibiotic resistant.

These, and the less common species of *Corynebacterium*, are described in a large review (36).

Coryneform bacteria, or "diphtheroids." Include many other species or groups that represent usual flora of skin and mucous membranes. Certain diphtheroids without species designations are becoming more prominent as opportunistic pathogens, e.g., Groups F-1, G.

Coxiella. *C. burnetii* is an obligate, intracellular, gram-negative bacterium of the family *Rickettsiaceae*. It is transmitted to many different animal species by ticks and results in Q fever. *C. burnetii* usually is transmitted to humans by inhalation of aerosol containing organisms (especially following parturition of an infected animal), by ingestion of raw milk or cheese, or rarely by tick bites. It is present in the United States in cattle, sheep, and goats. Clinical findings may include bronchopneumonia and, occasionally, liver granulomas and hepatitis, endocarditis, pericarditis, or meningitis (69). It may occur as an acute or chronic infection.

Delftia. *Delftia acidovorans* is a non-glucose-fermentative rod that was formerly classified as a *Pseudomonas* species. It is a hospital environmental organism that occasionally causes device-associated infections, including bacteremia.

Dermabacter. As the name implies, these gram-positive coryneform bacilli constitute part of the normal skin flora.

Dermatophilus congolensis. An actinomycete that causes dermatophilosis, a pustular dermatitis that heals by crusting and leaves some scarring. It usually affects animals and, rarely, humans. Humans become infected by contact with infected animals, such as cattle, sheep, horses, and goats.

DF-2. See *Capnocytophaga canimorsus.*

Diphtheroids. A general descriptive term applied to *Corynebacterium* species resembling *C. diphtheriae*. See *Corynebacterium*.

Diplococcus pneumoniae. See *Streptococcus pneumoniae*.

Döderlein's bacillus. See *Lactobacillus*.

Donovania granulomatis. See *Calymmatobacterium granulomatis*.

Dysgonomonas. Recently named genus of fastidious gram-negative bacilli similar to *Capnocytophaga*. *Dysgonomonas* has occasionally been recovered from the gallbladder or feces of patients with diarrhea.

Eaton agent. See *Mycoplasma pneumoniae*.

Edwardsiella tarda. Infrequently encountered species of gram-negative rods of the family *Enterobacteriaceae*. It appears to be part of the normal gastrointestinal flora of cold-blooded animals, and causes a *Salmonella*-like illness in humans. It has also been isolated from urine, abscesses, and infected tissues in cases of acute gastroenteritis, septicemia, osteomyelitis, and meningitis.

EF-4. CDC group EF-4 resembles *Kingella* spp., except that it is a part of the normal oral flora of dogs and cats, and thus a cause of bite-wound infections.

Ehrlichia. A genus of obligate intracellular (primarily leukocytes) bacteria closely related to rickettsiae. A cause of zoonotic infections most often transmitted by tick bites. The two species that infect humans are listed below. In addition, several other organisms previously classified as ehrlichiae now belong to the genera *Anaplasma* and *Neorickettsia*.

> *E. chaffeensis.* The cause of human monocyto-tropic ehrlichiosis (HME), a febrile illness characterized by high fever, malaise, myalgia, and, in about one-third of patients, a rash. Severe manifestations of the infection include a toxic shock-like syndrome or adult respiratory distress syndrome, in particular, in immunocompromised patients (63).

> *E. ewingii.* The cause of canine granulocytic ehrlichiosis, with a few cases reported in humans.

Eikenella. *E. corrodens* (formerly *Bacteroides corrodens,* HB-1) is a species of microaerophilic, non-glucose-fermentative, gram-negative rods. It is considered part of the normal mouth, genitourinary, and gastrointestinal flora. *E. corrodens* has been isolated from dental abscesses, from the bloodstream immediately after dental extractions, from wounds inflicted by human bites, and from pneumonia, empyema, otitis media, sinusitis, intra-abdominal infections, postoperative wound infections, septic arthritis, bacteremia, endocarditis, and meningitis. It is the "E" in the HACEK group of organisms (19).

Enterobacter **(formerly *Aerobacter*).** Genus of gram-negative rods of the family *Enterobacteriaceae*. It is present in soil, water, dairy products, and the human intestinal tract. Most infections in humans are hospital acquired.

E. aerogenes. Has caused urinary tract infections, pneumonia, surgical wound infections, bacteremia, endocarditis, and meningitis.

E. agglomerans. Now known as *Pantoea agglomerans*.

E. amnigenus. One of the newest species of this genus. It has caused wound and respiratory tract infections.

E. asburiae. Also a new species of *Enterobacter* that has caused urinary and respiratory tract infections and bacteremia.

E. cancerogenus. More recently known as *E. taylorae.*

E. cloacae. Has produced urinary tract infections, wound infections, pneumonia, bacteremia, and meningitis, and it is perhaps the most frequently isolated *Enterobacter* species. It is especially noted for its ability to produce a potent chromosomal β-lactamase that confers broad penicillin and cephalosporin resistance.

E. gergoviae. Has been isolated from urine, pulmonary infections, and bacteremia.

E. hafniae. See *Hafnia alvei.*

E. hormaechei. Is a recently named, uncommon member of this genus.

E. intermedius. Also a new, rarely encountered species.

E. liquefaciens. See *Serratia liquefaciens.*

E. sakazakii. Has been associated most notably with neonatal sepsis and meningitis.

Enterobacteriaceae. Very large family of facultative, glucose-fermentative, gram-negative bacilli that includes primarily the following genera that cause infections in humans: *Cedecea, Citrobacter, Edwardsiella, Enterobacter, Ewingella, Hafnia, Klebsiella, Kluyvera, Morganella, Pantoea, Proteus, Providencia, Salmonella, Serratia, Shigella, Tatumella,* and *Yersinia.*

Enterococcus. A genus of aerobic gram-positive cocci that were previously classified as species of bile-tolerant group D streptococci found in human and animal intestines. However, enterococci have been assigned their own genus, in part, due to their increasing clinical significance. They are among the most important causes of community- and hospital-acquired infections, including urinary tract infections, wound infections, bacteremia, endocarditis, and meningitis. They are much more resistant to anti-microbial agents than the so-called nonenterococcal group D streptococci (*S. bovis*) (38). There are now 22 recognized species of this important genus, but the most frequently encountered species are *E. faecalis* and *E. faecium.* Perhaps the most significant development in the genus has been the emergence in recent years of vancomycin resistance, most notably in *E. faecium* (27, 65, 72). In addition, two less-common species have an intrinsic "intermediate" level of susceptibility to vancomycin, i.e., *E. casseliflavus* and *E. gallinarum.*

Erwinia. See *Enterobacter agglomerans.*

Erysipelothrix rhusiopathiae. Species of facultative gram-positive rods that decolorize easily and may appear gram-negative. *E. rhusiopathiae* is primarily a pathogen of swine and turkeys. It causes erysipelas (erysipeloid) in animals and humans, a skin infection, particularly of the hands, with lymphadenopathy and, occasionally, arthritis. It has also produced rapidly fatal septicemia and endocarditis. Infections occur from direct contact with infected materials (meat, poultry, and hides). *Erysipelothrix* demonstrates intrinsic resistance to vancomycin, an unusual trait among gram-positive bacteria.

Escherichia. The most commonly encountered genus of facultative gram-negative rods of the family *Enterobacteriaceae.* It is widely distributed in nature and in animal and human intestinal tracts.

E. coli. Part of the normal human and animal intestinal flora and has often been used as an indicator of fecal contamination of water. It is the most frequent cause of human urinary tract infections (cystitis and pyelonephritis). It may also cause puerperal sepsis, cholecystitis, appendicitis, peritonitis, wound infections, pneumonia, empyema, bacteremia, endocarditis, meningitis, and at least four types of gastroenteritis [toxigenic diarrhea (diarrhea of travelers), hemorrhagic colitis (often due to serotype O157:H7), enteroinvasive diarrhea, and enteropathogenic disease in neonates]. *E. coli* O157:H7 is a notable cause of bloody diarrhea, and by virtue of producing Shiga toxin, may lead to the hemolytic-uremic syndrome (HUS) (79). Newer, but far less common, species include *E. fergusonii, E. hermannii,* and *E. vulneris.*

Eubacterium. Genus of anaerobic, non-spore-forming, gram-positive rods that have been isolated from soil, water, and animal and plant products. Occasional infections in humans have included wound infections, pulmonary infections, bacteremia, and various abscesses. This genus has undergone recent unfortunate taxonomic revision into a number of arcane genera, not further described here, of which many have been isolated from the human gingiva, but without evidence of disease production.

Facultative. The ability of a bacterium to grow in either aerobic or anaerobic atmospheres. Also called "facultative anaerobe."

Fastidious bacteria. Bacteria that require complex or enriched culture media for growth, often including blood or blood components. Examples include streptococci, *Haemophilus* species, the pathogenic

Neisseria species, *Pasteurella*, *Eikenella* species, *Capnocytophaga* species, and others.

Flavobacterium. Genus of yellow-pigmented, nonfermentative, gram-negative bacilli widely distributed in soil, water, and dairy products and occasionally isolated from debilitated patients. However, recent taxonomic changes have moved nearly all of the species associated with human infections to either the *Chryseobacterium*, *Empedobacter*, *Myroides*, or *Weeksella* genera.

Francisella tularensis (formerly *Pasteurella tularensis*). Species of aerobic, very small gram-negative coccobacilli that often show bipolar staining. *F. tularensis* has been isolated from many wild animals and insects and from human clinical specimens (local lesions, blood, sputum, gastric aspirates, conjunctival swabs, and pleural fluid). The cause of tularemia consists of three main categories, depending on the site of infection: (i) ulceroglandular tularemia, with a local skin lesion and regional lymphadenitis; (ii) oculoglandular, with conjunctivitis or conjunctival ulcer and regional lymphadenitis; or (iii) pulmonary, with pneumonitis. Bacteremia, toxemia, pharyngitis, and miliary necrosis to almost all organs may occur. It is transmitted to humans through handling of infected animals, by fleas, or via the respiratory or gastrointestinal tract. Infections have occasionally been traced to contaminated water. Recent taxonomic changes have resulted in *F. tularensis* being designated *F. tularensis* subsp. *tularensis*. Other close relatives with unclear clinical significance in humans include *F. tularensis* subsp. *holartica, F. tularensis* subsp. *novicida,* or *F. philomiragia. F. tularensis* has also been listed as a possible agent of bioterrorism.

Friedländer's bacillus. See *Klebsiella pneumoniae.*

Fusobacterium. Genus of anaerobic, spindle-shaped or otherwise pleomorphic, gram-negative rods often found in mixed infections with other anaerobes (32).

F. mortiferum. Has been cultured from the mouth and feces, from abscesses of the liver, and from persons with septicemia.

F. necrophorum. May be part of the normal flora of the mouth, intestinal tract, and genital tract. However, it has caused severe peritonsillar abscesses, neck abscesses, aspiration pneumonia, empyema, brain abscesses, septicemia, metastatic abscesses (Lemierre's disease), and septic thrombophlebitis.

F. nucleatum. Has been recovered from the mouth, and also from the genital and gastrointestinal tracts. The most commonly isolated *Fusobacterium* species, it is a cause of pulmonary infections, intra-abdominal infections, and bacteremia.

F. varium. Has been cultured from human feces, from clinical specimens, and from peritonitis and abdominal wounds.

Gaffkya. Genus of microaerophilic or anaerobic gram-positive cocci in tetrads. It is now classified as either *Peptococcus* or *Micrococcus.*

Gamma streptococci. Streptococci that produce no hemolysis on blood agar. A typical example is nonhemolytic *Streptococcus salivarius.*

Gardnerella vaginalis (**formerly** *Haemophilus vaginalis* **or** *Corynebacterium vaginale*). Species of facultative, fastidious, small, gram-variable, pleomorphic rods that appears to be part of the normal vaginal flora of many women. However, *G. vaginalis* is associated with bacterial vaginosis (nonspecific vaginitis along with *Mobiluncus* and *Campylobacter*). It may be seen on "clue cells" (epithelial cells covered with small gram-positive and gram-negative rods). It has also been isolated from amniotic fluid, endometrium, abdominal fluid, urine, and blood. It is a rare cause of bacteremia in women with postpartum fever or in infected neonates.

Gemella. Genus of gram-positive cocci or coccobacilli resembling some staphylococci or streptococci. They form part of the normal nasopharyngeal and skin microflora.

> **G. haemolysans.** Has been reported as a cause of endocarditis, meningitis, or prosthetic joint infections.

> **G. morbillorum (formerly *Streptococcus morbillorum*).** Has been isolated from respiratory tracts, genitourinary tracts, wound infections, and bacteremia.

Gonococcus. See *Neisseria gonorrhoeae.*

Gordonia. Genus of aerobic gram-positive, slightly branching rods resembling *Nocardia* spp. Usually associated with skin, or lung infections, or as a rare cause of bacteremia in immunosuppressed or debilitated patients.

Granulicatella. As with *Abiotrophia*, a relatively new genus composed of gram-positive cocci that were formerly referred to as "nutritionally deficient" or "satelliting" streptococci. These were originally considered to be nutritionally defective members of the viridans group of streptococci, then called *Abiotrophia* spp. However, the new genus contains two former *Abiotrophia* species, *G. adiacens* and *G. elegans*. These organisms are best known as occasional agents of endocarditis.

HACEK bacteria. Acronym for a group of genera of fastidious gram-negative bacilli that may cause bacteremia or endocarditis. They include *Haemophilus*, *Actinobacillus*, *Cardiobacterium*, *Eikenella*, and *Kingella* (19).

Haemophilus. Genus of fastidious, small, pleomorphic, gram-negative bacilli. Most members are part of the normal flora of the mucous membranes of the upper respiratory tract. Infections are more common in children than adults. *Haemophilus* species commonly cause otitis media, sinusitis, conjunctivitis, acute epiglottitis (croup), bronchitis, cellulitis, pneumonia, bacteremia, septic arthritis, osteomyelitis, and meningitis. Some species may also cause endocarditis.

H. aegyptius **(Koch-Weeks bacillus).** Causes a purulent and contagious conjunctivitis, especially in hot, tropical climates. It is largely indistinguishable from *H. influenzae*.

H. aphrophilus. Has been found in blood and pus and has caused endocarditis, meningitis, pneumonia, and empyema. It is the most frequent species of

Haemophilus to cause endocarditis, and is the "H" in the HACEK group (19).

H. ducreyi. The cause of chancroid (soft chancre). Transmitted by sexual contact, it is one of the most common sexually transmitted diseases in some developing countries, especially those with tropical or semitropical climates (e.g., Asia, Africa, Latin America).

H. haemolyticus. A part of the normal flora of the upper respiratory tract. It is a rare cause of endocarditis. It may morphologically resemble group A *Streptococcus* colonies when cultivated on some types of blood agar (but not on sheep blood agar).

H. influenzae (Pfeiffer's bacillus). Carried in the nasopharynx of many healthy individuals. Until an effective protein conjugate vaccine became available in 1992, *H. influenzae* type b was the most common cause of bacterial meningitis in young children. However, the use of the vaccine has largely eliminated it as a cause of meningitis in developed (but not developing) countries (64). Type b strains were also associated with acute epiglottitis and periorbital cellulitis. Encapsulated strains may also belong to serotypes a to f. In the postvaccine era, type f is the most common pathogenic serotype (78). Nonencapsulated strains continue to cause many cases of sinusitis, otitis media, bronchitis, conjunctivitis, septicemia, endocarditis, osteomyelitis, empyema, and pericarditis, and they often possess resistance mechanisms that affect commonly prescribed oral antibiotics (46). Certain biotypes of *H. influenzae* have recently been shown to cause serious urogenital and neonatal infections, including chorioamnionitis and bacteremia (37). The *H. influenzae* biogroup aegyptius causes a fulminant disease in children known as Brazilian purpuric fever (BPF).

H. parahaemolyticus. Normally may be found in the upper respiratory tract. It may be associated very rarely with endocarditis.

H. parainfluenzae. The most common *Haemophilus* species, which constitutes part of the normal flora of the upper respiratory tract. May also cause pneumonia, bacteremia, endocarditis, and very rarely meningitis.

H. paraphrophilus. Part of the normal oral microflora.

H. segnis. Part of the normal oral microflora.

H. vaginalis. Now named *Gardnerella vaginalis*.

Hafnia alvei (formerly *Enterobacter hafniae*). Species of gram-negative bacilli in the family *Enterobacteriaceae*. *H. alvei* has been associated with wound and respiratory and urinary tract infections, as well as being suggested as a rare cause of gastroenteritis.

Helicobacter. A diverse group of fastidious, microaerophilic, spiral-shaped gram-negative bacilli that inhabit the gastrointestinal tracts of many mammals and birds. They are closely related to *Campylobacter* species, and some members of that genus have been reclassified as species of *Helicobacter*. There are as many as 20 named species, although only one-third of that number has been recovered from humans.

   H. cinaedi and *H. fennelliae.* Have been implicated in cases of gastroenteritis (usually diarrhea) in immunocompromised individuals, especially those with AIDS (39).

   H. heilmanii. A much less common cause of gastritis, peptic ulcer disease, and gastrointestinal lymphomas.

   H. pylori. A prominent cause of gastric ulcer disease and cancers of the gastrointestinal tract. This striking cause-and-effect association was not widely acknowledged until the mid-1990s. Approximately 50% of the world's population is estimated to have *H. pylori* infection, making it one of the most common of all infectious diseases (60). The spectrum of disease ranges from asymptomatic infection to chronic atrophic gastritis.

Other *Helicobacter* species that have been associated with gastroenteritis or hepatobiliary disease include *H. canadensis, H. canis, H. pullorum, H. winghamensis*, and *H. bilis*.

Kingella. Genus of fastidious, coccoid to medium-sized, gram-negative rods with square ends that occur in pairs and short chains. *Kingella* spp. were previously classified as *Moraxella* spp. They are part of the normal oral and, possibly, genitourinary flora. *Kingella* spp. occasionally cause osteomyelitis, bacteremia, or endocarditis, and they are the "K" in HACEK (1, 19). Three main species of *Kingella* include *K. kingae, K. denitrificans*, and *K. oralis*.

Klebsiella. Genus of short, often plump, gram-negative rods of the family *Enterobacteriaceae*. *Klebsiella* has been isolated from humans, animals, water, and inanimate objects, and is part of the normal gastrointestinal flora. It is one of the most frequently clinically significant members of the enteric family.

K. ornithinolytica. May now also be known as *Raoutella ornithinolytica.* It is an uncommon cause of wound and urinary tract infections and bacteremia.

K. oxytoca. Produces disease similar to that caused by *K. pneumoniae,* and is the second most frequently isolated species of this genus.

K. ozaenae. Produces ozena, an atrophic, odiferous disease of the nasal mucosa, and other chronic upper respiratory tract infections. It has less commonly caused infections of the urinary tract, soft tissue, middle ear, and blood.

K. pneumoniae (Friedländer's bacillus). Part of the normal flora of the gastrointestinal tract and an occasional colonizer of the upper respiratory tract. It is a prominent cause of pneumonia, lung abscess, sinusitis, endocarditis, septicemia, meningitis, peritonitis, liver and biliary tract disease, wound infections, uterine and vaginal infections, salpingitis, osteomyelitis, and skin and urinary tract infections. Debilitated persons, alcoholics, and cirrhotics are especially susceptible to respiratory tract infections by this organism.

K. rhinoscleromatis. Produces rhinoscleroma, a chronic, destructive, granulomatous process of the nasopharynx. It is rare in the United States, but common in India, southeastern Europe, and Central America.

Kluyvera. A recently added genus of the family *Enterobacteriaceae.* It is rarely associated with serious human infections. Species include *K. ascorbata, K. cochleae, K. georgiana,* and *K. cryocrescens.*

Koch-Weeks bacillus. See *Haemophilus aegyptius.*

Kocuria. A genus of aerobic gram-positive cocci that is closely related to the genus *Micrococcus.* These cocci are normal skin inhabitants that very rarely cause disease.

Kurthia. A genus of aerobic gram-positive bacilli formerly classified with the corynebacteria. It has been isolated from the environment and from certain animals, but its role as a human pathogen is unproven.

Lactobacillus. Genus of microaerophilic or anaerobic gram-positive rods that represent part of the normal flora of the vagina, mouth, and intestinal tract. It plays an important role as normal flora in suppressing growth of pathogenic microorganisms in areas where they exist. Many species are widely distributed in dairy products, water, sewage, grains, meat products, and wines. It is a rare cause of human disease, such as pneumonia and bacteremia (6). Up to 90% of human isolates demonstrate intrinsic resistance to vancomycin.

Lactococcus. Genus of aerobic gram-positive cocci that share some phenotypic characteristics with *Enterococcus* spp., but rarely cause disease in humans.

Leclercia. An infrequently isolated genus of the family *Enterobacteriaceae*. It may cause pulmonary infections or bacteremia.

L forms. Bacteria devoid of a rigid cell wall (cell wall-defective bacteria). L forms theoretically may develop after exposure to cell wall-active antibiotics. Because they lack a cell wall, they may be able to resist conventional antibiotic therapy. They have been found among *Streptobacillus moniliformis, Haemophilus influenzae,* enteric bacilli, and streptococci, but their role, if any, in disease is unclear.

Legionella. Genus of aerobic, fastidious, very small, poorly staining, gram-negative bacilli found normally in water and soil. Various members have been recovered from streams, potable water supplies, plumbing pipes, hot water heaters, and air-conditioning cooling water (89). *Legionella* spp. are the cause of Legionnaires' disease, which is usually a severe atypical pneumonia. Special silver staining (Deiterle or Gimenez) is required for visualization in tissue because of poor gram-staining characteristics. Also, very specialized culture medium (Buffered Charcoal Yeast Extract) and several days' incubation are required for isolation. There has been a proliferation of named species of *Legionella* (now more than 40 species); however, most infections are caused by *L. pneumophila*, *L. micdadei*, *L. longbeachae*, *L. dumoffii*, and *L. bozemanii*. All the named species appear to be able to cause a type of Legionnaires' disease. The following species are most notable for historical reasons.

L. micdadei. Formerly TATLOCK, HEBA, or Pittsburgh pneumonia agent. Along with *L. pneumophila*, a prominent cause of pneumonia in immunosuppressed patients. May be hospital acquired from potable or hot water systems.

L. pneumophila. Now classic agent of Legionnaires' disease, or "Broad Street pneumonia," a febrile respiratory illness that may occur sporadically or in epidemics. It may also result in bacteremia and endocarditis. Transmission is airborne in water droplets, with no evidence of person-to-person spread.

Leprosy. See *Mycobacterium leprae*.

Leptospira. Genus of tightly coiled spirochetes that frequently appear with one bent end forming a hook. They are placed in "saprophytic" (*L. biflexa*) and "pathogenic" (*L. interrogans*) species. The saprophytic leptospires are normally present in fresh surface waters. The pathogens usually produce infection in animals (rats, mice, cattle, horses, hogs, wild rodents, goats, and dogs) and are excreted in the urine and feces, where they remain viable for several weeks. They may contaminate stagnant water or food supplies. Humans acquire infection from ingestion of contaminated sources or through skin breaks or mucous membranes. *Leptospira* spp. may spread to infect the liver, kidneys, central nervous system, skin, muscles, or eyes. They may occasionally be visualized in body fluids by dark-field microscopy or by means of special stains. Culture using specialized media is slow and complex. They may be isolated from blood, urine, or cerebrospinal fluid.

L. biflexa. A closely related species that can only be separated reliably by genotypic tests.

L. interrogans. Produces the most severe leptospiral infection, Weil's disease. It has worldwide distribution; the most common sources of infection are rat urine and contaminated water. It may also be hosted by dogs, mice, skunks, foxes, and raccoons. Its prevalence in rats may range up to 40%.

Leptotrichia. Genus of gram-negative anaerobes that is part of the normal flora of the mouth, intestine, and urogenital tract. It rarely causes disease.

Leuconostoc. Genus of aerobic gram-positive cocci that shares some phenotypic characteristics with *Enterococcus* spp., but only rarely causes disease in humans, such as wound infections, bacteremia, and meningitis. The most unique feature is its intrinsic resistance to vancomycin.

Listeria monocytogenes. Species of facultative, gram-positive, diphtheroid-like bacilli that may also appear coccobacillary. It has been found in soil and water and in animals and humans, where it has been isolated from the genital tract, nasopharynx, local lesions, meconium, feces, blood, and cerebrospinal fluid. *L. monocytogenes* is an important veterinary pathogen that causes abortion and encephalitis in sheep and cattle. It may cause an influenza-like illness in otherwise healthy women during pregnancy; this results in infection of the fetus, which leads to abortions, stillbirths, or neonatal septicemia and meningitis. Abscesses, skin lesions, upper respiratory tract infections, conjunctivitis, bacteremia, and meningitis may occur in immunocompromised adults or animal handlers. About half of all infections occur in neonates from symptomatic infected mothers. Infected pregnant women sometimes give a history of ingesting raw milk from cows or goats, soft cheeses, cole slaw, frankfurters, and smoked fish. In recent years, *Listeria* has been recognized as an important food-borne pathogen, giving rise to serious, sometimes fatal systemic disease in immunocompromised individuals (especially those with T-cell-mediated immune defects) who ingest contaminated food (58). The organism has the unique ability to proliferate in foods stored at refrigeration temperature.

Lyme disease. See *Borrelia burgdorferi.*

Meningococcus. See *Neisseria meningitidis.*

Methylobacterium. A recently created genus of pink-pigmented, non-glucose-fermentative, gram-negative bacilli. It is normally found on vegetation and in water (including tap water). *M. mesophilicum* (formerly *Pseudomonas mesophilica*) is the most common member of this genus to cause human infections (49). Most infections are associated with dialysis catheters, skin infections, or bacteremia.

Microbacterium. Aerobic gram-positive rod, similar to *Corynebacterium* spp. It is a rare cause of foreign body infections.

Micrococcaceae. Family of gram-positive cocci that includes *Micrococcus* and *Staphylococcus*.

Micrococcus. Genus of aerobic, saprophytic, gram-positive, coagulase-negative cocci from the family *Micrococcaceae*. It is widely distributed in nature and commonly found on human skin and mucous membranes; it only occasionally causes infections in humans, such as catheter-related bacteremia. Organisms formerly classified as *Micrococcus,* subgroups 1 through 4, have been reclassified as *Staphylococcus saprophyticus,* a common cause of urinary tract infections in young women (43).

Mima polymorpha. See *Acinetobacter calcoaceticus* var. *lwoffii.*

Mima polymorpha var. *oxidans.* See *Oligella urethralis.*

Mobiluncus. Highly motile, curved, irregular gram-positive (or gram-negative) staining anaerobic rods. They are frequently recovered from the vagina or rectum, and represent one of the microbial components responsible for bacterial vaginosis.

Moellerella. An infrequently encountered genus of the family *Enterobacteriaceae* that may cause opportunistic infections.

Mollicutes. Organisms that are smaller than conventional bacteria and lack the rigid cell wall of other bacteria, making them the smallest free-living organism known. *Mollicutes* includes the genera *Mycoplasma* and *Ureaplasma*.

Morax-Axenfeld bacillus. See *Moraxella lacunata*.

Moraxella. Genus of aerobic gram-negative cocci, coccobacilli, or diplobacilli. Some species represent normal flora of skin or mucous membranes of humans and certain animals. *Moraxella* contains a single species of gram-negative diplococci, *M. catarrhalis* (formerly *Branhamella catarrhalis* or *Neisseria catarrhalis*). *M. catarrhalis* is carried transiently as part of the normal nasopharyngeal flora, and colonizes a large percentage (>50%) of children. It is most notable as a cause of otitis media and sinusitis, but it can also cause acute bronchopulmonary infections, conjunctivitis, and less commonly, bacteremia, pericarditis, endocarditis, and meningitis (47). Several of the bacillary species of *Moraxella* are listed below.

M. atlantae. Part of the normal nasopharyngeal flora.

M. catarrhalis. Formerly *Branhamella catarrhalis* (see above).

M. lacunata (**Morax-Axenfeld bacillus**). Has been isolated from patients with conjunctivitis.

M. nonliquefaciens. Occasionally pathogenic and recovered from conjunctivitis, sinusitis, and bronchitis. It is part of the normal flora of the skin, nasopharynx, and genitourinary tract.

M. osloensis. Has been isolated rarely as an opportunistic pathogen. It is part of the normal flora of the skin, nasopharynx, and genitourinary tract.

Morganella morganii (**formerly *Proteus morganii***). Species of gram-negative rods of the family *Enterobacteriaceae*. It is closely related to *Proteus*. It may cause genitourinary tract infections, wound infections, bacteremia, meningitis, and a variety of other infectious processes. *M. morganii* is often resistant to a number of the most commonly used antimicrobial agents.

MRSA. Acronym for methicillin-resistant *Staphylococcus aureus* (see below).

Mycobacterium. Genus of relatively slow-growing bacilli characterized by acid-fast staining but poor gram-staining characteristics. *Mycobacterium* contains both saprophytic and pathogenic species. "Anonymous," "Atypical," or "Unclassified" mycobacteria are old designations for *Mycobacterium* species other than *M. tuberculosis* (MOTT). Many are inhabitants of soil or water, but some are notable human pathogens.

Runyan groups I to IV. Represent an historical means of classifying mycobacteria other than *M. tuberculosis* on the basis of colony pigmentation and in vitro growth rate.

Group I. Photochromogens. Produce little or no pigment when grown in the dark but yellow-orange pigments after brief exposure to light. Growth may be slightly faster than that of *M. tuberculosis*.

Group II. Scotochromogens. Produce pigment

when grown in either dark or light.

Group III. Nonphotochromogens. Produce light-tan colonies without pigment.

Group IV. Rapid growers. Usually grow within 3 to 10 days on routine laboratory media.

The most common *Mycobacterium* species include:

***M. abscessus* (formerly *M. chelonei* subsp. *abscessus*).** One of the most common and most pathogenic of the rapidly growing *M. fortuitum* complex (90). It is an important cause of chronic lung disease (90% of those that are due to rapidly growing mycobacteria), posttraumatic wound infections, and posttympanostomy tube otitis media. It is also a cause of disseminated cutaneous infections, mammoplasty wound infections, sternal wound infections, and catheter-associated bacteremia. Its natural habitat may be tap water.

M. africanum. A close relative of *M. tuberculosis* and a cause of tuberculosis in tropical Africa.

M. asiaticum. A rare cause of pulmonary infections reported from Australia and the United States, as well as joint infections.

M. avium. A nonphotochromogen originally isolated from birds. It causes avian tuberculosis in fowl, cattle, swine, and humans. A very important cause of disseminated disease in immunosuppressed patients, such as those with AIDS (44). *M. avium* is often not distinguished from *M. intracellulare,* a closely related species.

Battey bacillus. See *M. intracellulare.*

M. bovis. Produces a progressive pulmonary disease in humans and many warm-blooded animals that is indistinguishable from tuberculosis caused by *M. tuberculosis,* although it sometimes is less virulent. Now rare in the United States, it can be acquired by ingestion of infected unpasteurized milk. Bacillus Calmette-Guérin (BCG) is an attenuated strain of *M. bovis* used for vaccine preparation in some parts of the world.

M. canetti. The most recently described member of the *M. tuberculosis* complex. It has caused generalized lymphadenitis and tuberculosis in patients with AIDS in Africa.

M. celatum. A slow-growing nonphotochromogen that has caused rare pulmonary infections, especially in patients with AIDS.

M. chelonei (formerly *M. chelonei* subsp. *chelonei*). May be the second most pathogenic member of the *M. fortuitum* complex. It is slower growing than other members of the group. It is most often a cause of serious, disseminated nodular skin disease in immunosuppressed patients, and an important cause of posttraumatic skin infections and catheter infections.

M. conspicuum. A slowly growing organism isolated originally from patients with AIDS.

M. flavescens. A scotochromogen of very low virulence.

M. fortuitum. Has been isolated from water and soil. It is often associated with clusters of nosocomial infections, most often, surgical wound infections, cellulitis, otitis media, and rarely chronic pulmonary infections.

M. fortuitum-complex. An historical classification that has included *M. abscessus*, *M. chelonei*, and *M. fortuitum*.

M. fortuitum-group. Now refers to closely related organisms that are difficult to separate by phenotypic tests, and includes *M. fortuitum*, *M. peregrinum*, and two other unnamed biovariants.

M. gastri. A slow-growing nonphotochromogen rarely associated with disease in humans. It is isolated from gastric washings, sputum, and soil.

M. genavense. Is the most common cause of mycobacterial disease in psittacine birds, and causes an *M. avium*-like infection in patients with AIDS.

M. gordonae (tap-water scotochromogen). Has frequently been cultured from tap water, soil, sputum, and gastric lavage specimens, but it rarely causes disease.

M. haemophilum. Slow-growing nonchromogen that requires hemin or complex iron-supplemented media, as well as cooler incubation temperatures (e.g., 30 to 32°C) for growth. It is isolated primarily from ulcerating skin lesions of immuno-suppressed patients, especially those with AIDS (21), and occasionally associated with cervical lymphadenopathy in children.

M. interjectum. A scotochromogen recovered rarely from children with lymphadenitis.

M. intracellulare (formerly Battey bacillus). A group III nonphotochromogen originally isolated from lymph nodes and in cases of a pulmonary disease indistinguishable from tuberculosis.

M. intracellulare may not be readily distinguished from *M. avium*. Members of the *M. avium-intracellulare* complex (MAC) produce serious disseminated infections in patients with AIDS.

M. kansasii. A photochromogen that in humans produces a pulmonary disease sometimes indistinguishable from that caused by *M. tuberculosis.* May also produce cervical and hilar lymphadenopathy, bone infections, cutaneous and soft-tissue infections. Its natural reservoir appears to be tap water. It is the second most commonly isolated MOTT (30).

M. lentiflavum. A slow-growing, pigmented organism from respiratory specimens.

***M. leprae* (Hansen's bacillus).** The causative agent of leprosy. Has not as yet been cultivated on artificial laboratory media, but has been cultured in the foot pads of mice. May be seen as acid-fast organisms in parallel aggregates on smears or in biopsies of skin, nasal mucosa, and other tissues (9).

M. malmoense. A nonphotochromogen that is very slow growing, and has been isolated as an occasional cause of cervical lymphadenitis in children or from chronic pulmonary infection in adults in northern Europe.

M. marinum (formerly *M. balnei*). A photo-chromogen originally isolated from tuberculous lesions of saltwater fish. Produces epidemic or chronic skin lesions (swimming-pool granulomas) and sporotrichoid mycobacteriosis in humans. It often requires incubation at cooler temperatures (30 to 32°C) for reliable recovery.

M. microti. A cause of tuberculosis in a variety of warm-blooded animals, and it has infected occasional immunosuppressed and immunocompetent humans. So far, it has not been cultivated successfully in vitro.

M. mucogenicum. A nonpigmented rapid grower that can be easily recovered from tap water. It is an occasional cause of soft-tissue infection, catheter sepsis, or pulmonary infection.

M. phlei. Found in nature and on human skin. It very rarely produces disease.

M. scrofulaceum. A scotochromogen that produces suppurative cervical adenitis in young children. It has been isolated infrequently from lung tissue, sputum, and lymph nodes.

M. shimoidei. A very rare cause of pulmonary infections in humans.

M. simiae. Originally isolated from monkeys, but more recently shown to cause chronic pulmonary disease in humans.

M. smegmatis. A rapidly growing organism originally recovered from human smegma. However, it is an occasional cause of soft-tissue infections following surgery or trauma.

M. szulgai. A scotochromogen that has produced pulmonary infections similar to those of tuberculosis, and occasional soft-tissue or joint infections.

M. terrae. A slow-growing nonphotochromogen that has caused rare extrapulmonary disease. It is isolated from soil and water.

M. triplex. A slow-growing, nonpigmented organism that resembles *M. avium.* It has been recovered from lymph nodes and respiratory specimens.

M. triviale. Currently a member of the *M. terrae* complex. It is a nonchromogen that rarely causes disease in humans.

M. tuberculosis. The causative agent of tuberculosis. It enters the body via the respiratory tract, by ingestion, or through the skin. Lesions may involve almost every organ of the body, but most commonly the lungs. *M. tuberculosis* continues to be a pathogen of major concern throughout the world.

M. ulcerans. Produces a chronic and deforming skin ulcer ("Buruli ulcer") in Africa and in certain other tropical areas. Its incidence may be underestimated because the organism is very difficult to cultivate in vitro.

M. xenopi. A nonphotochromogen that produces chronic pulmonary disease and occasional disseminated infections. Because it is a thermophilic organism that grows best at 42 to 45°C, it has been recovered from hot-water systems in hospitals during nosocomial clusters.

MOTT. Acronym for mycobacteria other than *M. tuberculosis.*

***Mycoplasma* (formerly pleuropneumonia-like organisms, or PPLO).** Genus of highly pleomorphic, very small, gram-negative bacteria lacking a cell wall. Cannot be seen on routine smears or in cultures on routine laboratory media. They normally reside on the mucous membranes of the respiratory and genitourinary tracts. Various species (described below) have been recovered during disease states from the lung, pleural fluid, blood, and joints (34). Several less common *Mycoplasma* species have been isolated from humans but have not proved to be the cause of human disease. Some strains (formerly called T strains) are now classified as *Ureaplasma urealyticum* (83).

M. fermentans. An apparent cause of lower respiratory tract infection in children and young adults.

M. genitalium. A recently described cause of cervicitis and pelvic inflammatory disease.

M. hominis. Can be isolated from the lower genital tracts of sexually active adults, but conclusive evidence that it causes urethritis in men or women has been hard to come by. It may, however, contribute to the process of bacterial vaginosis, and it rarely causes salpingitis and pyelonephritis. In addition, *M. hominis* has been isolated from the blood of immunosuppressed patients and of febrile women following septic abortion or normal deliveries. *M. hominis* has been recovered from the synovial fluids of persons with rheumatoid arthritis, stimulating a lively debate regarding its true etiology in this condition.

M. penetrans. A recently described species that at first was thought to cause a systemic infection in patients with AIDS, although firm evidence for that is lacking.

M. pneumoniae (formerly "Eaton agent pneumonia"). Causes approximately 20% of community-acquired pneumonia, often referred to as atypical pneumonia (34). *M. pneumoniae* infection often begins as tracheobronchitis or as an upper respiratory tract infection that may then progress to pneumonia in about one-third of the infections. Extrapulmonary complications, including meningoencephalitis, transverse myelitis, ascending paralysis, arthritis, and pericarditis occur occasionally. Nonspecific serologic reactions to infection by this agent include high titers of cold agglutinins in about half of infected persons.

Myroides. A genus of non-glucose-fermentative, gram-negative bacilli that was previously included in the *Flavobacterium* genus. Two current species are *M. odoratum* and *M. odoratimimus*, both of which are associated with moist areas of the hospital environment, and which can result in nosocomial infections, including wound infections, urinary tract infections, pneumonia, and bacteremia.

Neisseria. Genus of aerobic gram-negative cocci usually appearing in pairs with their sides flattened so that they have a "coffee-bean" appearance. Most members of the genus are commensals that inhabit the oropharynx and nasopharynx of humans. Only two species are considered frank human pathogens, *N. gonorrhoeae* and *N. meningitidis.*

   N. catarrhalis. See *Moraxella catarrhalis.*

   N. cinerea. Part of the normal oropharyngeal, genitourinary, and, possibly, gastrointestinal flora. It may be misidentified as *N. gonorrhoeae* by some laboratory methods.

   N. elongata. Part of the normal nasopharyngeal flora, but it has rarely been recovered from infections at other sites.

   N. gonorrhoeae (**gonococcus**). The etiologic agent of the sexually transmitted disease gonorrhea and may cause urethritis, cervicitis, vulvovaginitis, salpingitis, prostatitis, stomatitis, conjunctivitis, pharyngitis, epididymitis, bartholinitis, skin le-sions, arthritis, tenosynovitis, proctitis, septicemia, endocarditis, and ophthalmia of the newborn. It continues to be one of the most common sexually transmitted diseases in developed and developing countries.

N. *lactamica*. Regarded as part of the normal flora of the nasopharynx and throat. It has also been isolated from the urogenital tract, and it may resemble *N. meningitidis* in some laboratory identification tests.

N. *meningitidis* (meningococcus). Can transiently colonize the nasopharynx of asymptomatic carriers, where it may serve as the source of later infection. It is a prominent cause of meningitis, both endemic and epidemic. Epidemics have occurred among teenagers and young adults living in close proximity or having salivary contact. Military recruits are now routinely vaccinated against the four most common serogroups of meningococcus. Purpuric skin lesions may also develop during bacteremia (meningococcemia) or meningitis, and hemorrhage and necrosis of the adrenal glands may result in the Waterhouse-Friderichsen syndrome. *N. meningitidis* may also cause pneumonia, pericarditis, arthritis, osteomyelitis, and endophthalmitis. It has also been isolated from the genitourinary tract and anal canal.

N. flavescens, N. mucosa, N. polysaccharea, N. sicca, and *N. subflava.* Part of the normal nasopharyngeal flora and not normally a cause of disease.

Neorickettsia. Neorickettsia sennetsu is an obligate intracellular bacterium formerly classified as an *Ehrlichia* species. It is the cause of Sennetsu fever, a self-limited febrile illness that has occurred primarily in Japan. It is thought to be contracted from consumption of fluke-infested fish.

Nocardia. Genus of aerobic gram-positive, branching, filamentous bacteria. Some species are weakly or partially acid-fast. They are members of the large group of aerobic actinomycetes. Their normal habitat is soil and fresh and marine waters. They primarily cause infections in persons who are immunocompromised or through soft-tissue injury. The organism is acquired either through inhalation or through direct introduction by trauma. *N. asteroides* is the species responsible for the majority of serious invasive infections (55, 62).

N. abscessus. A recently described species involved with abscesses of the lower extremities.

N. asteroides. An opportunist that produces disease in persons with neoplasms or other immunosuppressive states, e.g., AIDS, organ transplant recipients, and those receiving systemic steroids (87). In these severely immunocompromised patients, invasive pulmonary disease often precedes systemic infection with resultant bacteremia, endocarditis, meningitis, cerebral abscess, kidney abscess, and lesions of the liver, skin, and lymph nodes. Cutaneous or ocular infections may occur in immunocompetent individuals following direct inoculation with soil or water. Cutaneous infections may present as chronic, suppurating granulomas with draining sinuses that discharge pigmented "sulfur" granules on the extremities, which may spread to regional lymph nodes, causing a lymphocutaneous syndrome.

N. brasiliensis. The predominant cause of actinomycetoma in North and South America, Mexico, and Australia. It is a cause of chronic subcutaneous abscesses (mycetomas), skin ulcers, and lymphocutaneous lesions resembling those of sporotrichosis. Lesions may extend to bone. Most often these infections occur on the lower extremities from walking barefooted (Madura foot). *N. brasiliensis* occasionally causes disseminated infection in immunocompromised patients.

N. caviae. Now known as *N. otitidiscaviarum.*

N. farcinica. Can cause a variety of cutaneous and systemic infections, including cerebral abscess, bacteremia, and kidney and pulmonary abscesses. It may be more virulent than N. *asteroides*, and is the most antibiotic-resistant member of the genus *Nocardia* (91).

N. nova. Appears to cause a number of different types of infections similar to those produced by N. *farcinica*.

N. otitidiscaviarum. Causes primarily cutaneous or ocular infections.

N. pseudobrasiliensis. Appears to cause pulmonary, central nervous system, and disseminated infections, as opposed to cutaneous infections.

N. transvalensis. A newly named species that may cause mycetoma as well as invasive pulmonary and disseminated infections.

N. africana, N. paucivorans, and **N. veterana.** Other newer or less common *Nocardia* species.

Nocardiopsis. A recently named genus of gram-positive bacteria that includes N. *dassonvillei*, a rare cause of mycetomas, and other skin infections. It includes six other even less common relatives of the genus *Nocardia*.

Nosocomial. Refers to an infection that is acquired in the hospital or as a result of medical care. Usually defined as occurring 48 hours or more following admission to a hospital or treatment in an outpatient setting.

Ochrobacterium. A genus of uncommonly occurring, aerobic gram-negative rods formerly classified as *Achromobacter* species of CDC group Vd. It is an environmental organism that occasionally causes catheter-related bacteremia. *O. anthropi* is the most frequently isolated species of *Ochrobacterium*.

Oerskovia. A genus of aerobic gram-positive coccoid to rod-shaped bacteria that occasionally are associated with foreign-body infections and bacteremia.

Oligella. This genus of uncommon gram-negative bacilli includes two species, *O. urethralis* (formerly *Moraxella urethralis* or before that, *Mima polymorpha* var. *oxidans*) and *O. urealytica* (formerly CDC group IVe), which represent part of the normal genitourinary flora and may rarely cause urinary tract infections.

Opportunist. An organism that is a member of the normal or transient body flora and is usually regarded as harmless in a specific location. This organism may produce disease if introduced into a normally sterile part of the body or if predisposing factors, such as neoplasm, trauma, or immunosuppression, are present.

Pantoea. A genus with one primary species infecting humans (*P. agglomerans*; formerly known as *Enterobacter agglomerans*), and thus a member of the family *Enterobacteriaceae*. An organism found in the hospital environment that may cause a variety of nosocomial infections, including wound infections, urinary tract infections, bacteremia, meningitis, brain abscess, and, historically, septicemia from contaminated intravenous fluids.

Pasteurella. Genus of aerobic, small, gram-negative rods or coccobacilli that may stain bipolarly. The natural reservoir is the nasopharynx and gingiva of various animals, although some species can cause hemorrhagic septicemia in some animal species. *Pasteurella* can produce serious disease in humans, with infection being transmitted by bites, scratches, or perhaps inhalation (35, 42).

P. bettyae **(formerly CDC group HB-5).** A rare cause of serious and localized infections in humans, but its normal animal reservoir remains unknown.

P. canis. An occasional cause of dog-bite wound infections.

P. dagmatis. A cause of cat- or dog-bite wound infections.

P. gallinarum. Occurs primarily in poultry, but it has caused rare cases of bacteremia in humans.

P. haemolytica. Causes infections primarily in cattle and sheep. Infections in humans have been very rare, but associated with animal exposure.

P. multocida. Part of the normal respiratory flora of cats, dogs, rats, rabbits, fowl, sheep, cattle, horses, and swine. It may infect humans after a scratch or bite by an animal carrying the organism or after exposure to the carcasses of infected animals. Following animal bites (particularly cat or dog bites), the infection can progress to septic arthritis, osteomyelitis, bacteremia, endocarditis, meningitis, pulmonary infection, liver abscess, pyelonephritis, or brain abscess. It is also possible for infection to begin with pulmonary disease following upper respiratory tract colonization for some period of time. It is the most frequently isolated *Pasteurella* species in humans.

P. pestis. Now known as *Yersinia pestis*.

P. pneumotropica. Thought to be part of the normal oral flora of rats, mice, and hamsters; it may infect humans through the bites of these animals and results in local infections. More recent information suggests that these strains may have been *P. dagmatis* instead.

P. pseudotuberculosis. Now known as *Yersinia pseudotuberculosis*.

P. stomatis. Associated with cat- or dog-bite infections.

P. ureae. Now known as *Actinobacillus ureae*.

PCR. Acronym for polymerase chain reaction, a patented technique for amplifying specific segments of DNA or RNA extracted from clinical specimens or cultures, so that the specific nucleic acid sequences can be used to detect or identify microorganisms or tumors, or establish parentage. Several other technologies also exist for accomplishing the amplification of nucleic acids, e.g., ligase chain reaction (LCR), strand displacement amplification (SDA), and transcription-mediated amplification (TMA). These procedures hold the promise of supplementing or replacing conventional culture and microscopy for diagnosis of infectious diseases.

Pediococcus. Genus of gram-positive cocci related to streptococci and enteroccci. *Pediococcus* is a very rare cause of septicemia and liver abscess in immunocompromised patients, and it is perhaps best known as one of several unusual gram-positive organisms with intrinsic resistance to vancomycin that could be confused with vancomycin-resistant *Enterococcus* species.

Peptococcus niger. Species of anaerobic gram-positive cocci. It is part of the normal flora of the oropharynx and genitourinary tract. It occasionally (along with other anaerobes) causes abscesses, particularly of the head, neck, and female genital tract. *P. niger* is the only currently recognized species of this genus.

Peptostreptococcus. Genus of the most frequently encountered anaerobic gram-positive cocci that may be cultured from the female genital tract, the mouth, and the upper respiratory and intestinal tracts. These "anaerobic streptococci" have been isolated from pelvic and appendiceal abscesses, infected sinuses and ears, gangrenous wounds, osteomyelitis, and bacteremia (32). Pathogenic species have included

P. magnus, P. tetradius, P. asaccharolyticus, P. anaerobius, P. micros, and *P. prevotii.* Unfortunately, molecular taxonomists have recently turned their attention to this genus, with the result that many of these species have been given new genus designations. These now include *Anaerococcus, Gallicola, Micromonas, Finegoldia, Schleiferella,* while still retaining three species of *Peptostreptococcus.* The clinician should simply regard this group as peptostreptococci or simply anaerobic streptococci.

Pertussis. See *Bordetella pertussis.*

Pfeiffer's bacillus. See *Haemophilus influenzae.*

Photorhabdus luminescens. Species of the family *Enterobacteriaceae* that was previously classified as *Xenorhabdus luminescens. P. luminescens* infects the larvae of some insects and rarely may cause wound infections and bacteremia in humans (31).

Pittsburgh pneumonia agent. See *Legionella micdadei.*

Plesiomonas shigelloides (formerly *Aeromonas shigelloides*). Species of aerobic gram-negative bacilli that are normally found in fresh and estuarine waters and the gastrointestinal tracts of a number of warm- and cold-blooded animals. *P. shigelloides* has been isolated from stools of asymptomatic as well as diarrheic persons. It also has been isolated from wound infections and from blood and cerebrospinal fluid. It was originally found in association with *Shigella* gastroenteritis and dysentery.

Pleuropneumonia-like organisms. See *Mycoplasma*.

Pneumococcus. See *Streptococcus pneumoniae*.

Porphyromonas. Genus of anaerobic gram-negative bacilli, many of which were previously classified as members of the genus *Bacteroides*. Several members of the genus produce darkly pigmented colonies following prolonged incubation on culture media. *Porphyromonas* species can be found in the normal flora of the oral cavity, and in some cases, also the urogenital and gastrointestinal tracts.

> *P. asaccharolyticus.* May cause lung abscesses, empyema, bite-wound infections, and infections of the urogenital and intestinal tracts. Other members of the genus (*P. gingivalis, P. endodontalis*) are involved in dental, oral, bite-wound, head and neck, and occasionally abdominal infections.

> *P. dentalis, P. gingivalis,* **and** *P. endodontalis.* Cause of periodontal and root canal abscesses.

PPLO (pleuropneumonia-like organisms). See *Mycoplasma*.

Prevotella. Genus of anaerobic gram-negative bacilli, many of which were previously classified as members of the genus *Bacteroides*. Members of the normal oral and, in some cases, genitourinary or intestinal flora of humans.

P. bivia (**previously** *Bacteroides bivius*). Part of normal urethral and vaginal flora, but now is also recognized as an important cause of various gynecologic and oral infections.

P. disiens (**previously** *Bacteroides disiens*). Also part of normal female genital tract flora, but also recognized as an important cause of gynecologic and oral infections.

P. leoscheii **and** *P. melaninogenica.* Part of the normal oral flora, but may cause oral or dental infections.

P. oris **and** *P. buccae.* Part of the normal oral flora and can be found in a variety of oral or pulmonary infections.

Propionibacterium. Genus of anaerobic, pleomorphic gram-positive rods that have been isolated from the human skin, mucous membranes, and intestinal tract.

P. acnes (formerly *Corynebacterium acnes*). Part of the normal skin flora. The acknowledged role of this species is with acne vulgaris pustules. It has been cultured from clinical specimens in cases of blepharitis, lung infection, abscesses, wounds, septicemia, endocarditis, and infected prosthetic devices (including cerebrospinal fluid shunts). Infections are often linked to surgical procedures or foreign bodies.

P. propionicum. May cause lacrimal duct infections.

P. avidum and *P. granulosum.* Less frequently encountered species that occasionally cause disease in humans.

Proteus. Genus of gram-negative rods from the family *Enterobacteriaceae,* some of which swarm on the surface of laboratory culture media. They may be found in soil, water, and sewage. These organisms are part of the normal fecal flora but may produce various infections when introduced into other sites. They are among the more commonly isolated members of the enteric group. They may cause chronic urinary tract infections (often with calculi), pneumonia, wound infections, bacteremia, and meningitis.

P. mirabilis. The *Proteus* species most frequently isolated from human sources. It is indole-negative and often susceptible to ampicillin. *P. mirabilis* has been isolated from urine, sputum, wounds, intra-abdominal abscesses, blood, and cerebrospinal fluid.

P. morganii. Now known as *Morganella morganii.*

P. penneri. A recently recognized species that may cause urinary tract or systemic infections.

P. rettgeri. Now known as *Providencia rettgeri.*

P. vulgaris. May be present as normal fecal flora, but it is also an opportunist occasionally isolated from urine, wounds, and blood.

Protoplasts. Cell wall-deficient microorganisms (usually of gram-positive bacilli), which are spherical and osmotically fragile. They differ from spheroplasts, which contain some cell wall material (although defective). They are of uncertain clinical significance.

Providencia. Genus of gram-negative rods of the family *Enterobacteriaceae* that are somewhat similar in biochemical activity to *Proteus*. Commonly present in feces, *Providencia* species include *P. alcalifaciens*, *P. hembachae*, *P. rettgeri*, *P. rustigiani*, and *P. stuartii*. They produce infections primarily in debilitated hosts, in particular, urinary tract infections, pneumonia, postoperative and burn-wound infections, hospital-acquired septicemia, and meningitis.

Pseudomonas. Genus of aerobic, non-glucose-fermentative, gram-negative rods. Several species produce visible or fluorescent green pigments. They are widely distributed in nature in soil, water, and vegetable matter. Many species are plant pathogens, but some cause infections in humans (predominantly in debilitated individuals, such as those with neoplasms, severe burns, or immunosuppression or on prolonged broad-spectrum antimicrobial therapy). They may contaminate various aqueous solutions and environments within healthcare institutions, and cause various nosocomial infections. They are the most commonly isolated gram-negative rods that are not members of the *Enterobacteriaceae*.

P. acidovorans (formerly ***Comamonas terrigena***). A common soil saprophyte that is occasionally found in clinical specimens, such as urine and sputum, and contaminated intravenous tubing.

P. aeruginosa. Has worldwide distribution. It is a common inhabitant of soil and water and the most common *Pseudomonas* species causing human infections. Pigment production varies; it is typically green and iridescent but may be bluish, brown, pink, or nonpigmented. *P. aeruginosa* is frequently present as part of the normal intestinal and skin flora. Because of its ability to survive in moist environments, it can be easily found in the hospital environment (e.g., in sinks, drains, soap solutions, disinfectants, dialysis fluids, whirlpools, respiratory therapy equipment, etc.). It may infect wounds (in which it produces thick blue-green pus) and may cause urinary tract infections (usually after instrumentation or catheterization), necrotizing pneumonia, empyema, otitis externa, eye infections (especially after surgery or injury), folliculitis (including that obtained from "hot tubs"), septicemia, endocarditis, and meningitis (12). *P. aeruginosa* often contaminates burns, draining wound sinuses, and decubitus ulcers. Infections are more likely to develop in immunosuppressed patients or those receiving antibiotics due to the broad, intrinsic resistance of this species to many commonly prescribed antibiotics.

P. alcaligenes. Has been recovered from swimming pools, rivers, fish, various animals, and human feces. It has been incriminated in urinary tract infections, respiratory tract infections, septicemia, and endocarditis.

P. fluorescens. A common inhabitant of soil and water, and perhaps human skin. It has been cultured from blood stored for transfusion, from contact lens solutions, from disinfectant solutions, and from pleural fluid, urine, sputum, nose, throat, wounds, and blood.

P. luteola. A rare cause of bacteremia, wound infection, or meningitis.

P. mallei. Now known as *Burkholderia mallei.*

P. maltophilia. Now known as *Stenotrophomonas maltophilia.*

P. mendocina. A very rare cause of infections in humans, primarily bacteremia and endocarditis.

P. oryzihabitans. A recently described species noted for causing catheter-related bacteremia, peritonitis in patients on chronic peritoneal dialysis, cellulitis and wound infections, and meningitis after neurosurgery.

P. pseudomallei. Now known as *Burkholderia pseudomallei.*

P. putida. A common inhabitant of soil, water, and plants. It is occasionally isolated from contact lens solutions, urine, and wounds, and it is known as a cause of catheter-related bacteremia.

P. stutzeri. A common soil and water saprophyte, but is occasionally encountered in clinical specimens, such as urine, sputum, wounds, ear drainage, and infected eyes, and in aerosolization equipment and contaminated dialyzers.

Psittacosis. See *Chlamydia psittaci.*

Psychrobacter. *Psychrobacter phenylpyruvica* is a non-glucose-fermentative, gram-negative rod that was formerly classified as *Moraxella phenylpyruvica*. It is an uncommon cause of ocular infections, bacteremia, and endocarditis.

Q-fever. See *Coxiella burnetii.*

Ralstonia. *Ralstonia pickettii* is a former *Pseudomonas* species that is an infrequent cause of a variety of infections, including bacteremia, endocarditis, and meningitis. It has caused nosocomial outbreaks due to contaminated solutions in a hospital setting. Little is known about several other recently described members of the genus.

Rhizobium. A recently named genus of aerobic gram-negative bacilli previously called *Agrobacterium.* *Rhizobium* species are principally plant pathogens that occasionally cause catheter-associated urinary tract, dialysis, or bloodstream infections. The most common species appears to be *R. radiobacter.*

Rhodococcus. Genus of aerobic, pleomorphic, gram-positive bacilli previously classified as either *Nocardia* or *Corynebacterium* species. It is normally found in soil and water and associated with livestock (particularly *R. equi* as a cause of disease in foals). *Rhodococcus* usually demonstrates salmon-pink- or orange-pigmented colonies in culture. It is a cause of disease in humans, primarily skin infections or granulomatous pneumonia in immunosuppressed individuals such as those with AIDS (23).

Rickettsia. Genus of minute, gram-negative, obligate, intracellular coccobacilli that are transmitted by arthropods and produce systemic diseases characterized most often by rash and fever.

R. africae. The cause of African tick bite fever. As implied, it is transmitted by tick bites in eastern and southern Africa and the Caribbean.

R. akari. The etiologic agent of rickettsial pox, which occurs in the northern United States,

Ukraine, Croatia, and Korea. It is often a mild disease characterized by a chickenpox-like rash and fever. Transmission is by mite bites, with the initial inoculation site developing into a black eschar. The natural reservoir is mice.

R. australis. Produces Queensland tick typhus in Australia. The reservoir is marsupials, and transmission is by tick bites.

R. conorii. The agent of Mediterranean fever (boutonneuse fever) in southern Europe, Africa, and the Middle East. The reservoir includes dogs and rodents, and transmission is via tick bites.

R. felis. The cause of cat flea typhus in the United States. It appears to be transmitted by flea bites.

R. honei. Causes Flinders Island spotted fever in Australia. It is transmitted by tick bites.

R. japonica. The cause of Japanese spotted fever. It is transmitted by tick bites.

R. prowazekii. Occurs worldwide. Transmitted by lice, it is the agent of epidemic typhus (classic louse-borne typhus), which is characterized by fever, prostration, and rash starting on the trunk region. A recrudescence of this disease is called "Brill-

Zinsser disease." The reservoir includes humans and flying squirrels.

R. rickettsii. Causes Rocky Mountain spotted fever in the Western Hemisphere. Transmission is by tick bites, and the reservoir includes deer, dogs, rodents, foxes, and humans. The rash starts peripherally, in contrast to that of epidemic and endemic typhus.

R. sibirica. Produces North Asian tick-borne typhus, a mild form of spotted fever. The reservoir is rodents, and transmission is by ticks.

R. tsutsugamushi (**now may be known as** *Orientia tsutsugamushi*). Causes scrub typhus (tsutsugamushi fever), clinically resembling epidemic typhus. It is transmitted by chigger mite bite; the site of the bite becomes a black eschar. The reservoir is rodents in Japan, eastern Asia, northern Australia, and the South and West Pacific.

R. typhi. Occurs worldwide and causes endemic (murine) typhus, which tends to be similar to, but milder than epidemic typhus. The reservoir is rats or other rodents, and transmission is by fleas.

Rochalimaea. See *Bartonella.*

Roseomonas. A new genus composed of pink-pigmented, aerobic, gram-negative bacilli. It includes the species *R. gilardi*, *R. cervicalis*, and *R. fauriae*. It is an infrequent cause of wound infections, bacteremia, urinary tract, and peritoneal dialysis infections (82).

Rothia. A genus of aerobic, pleomorphic, gram-positive rods, similar in morphology to corynebacteria. It occasionally causes lower respiratory tract infections or bacteremia.

Salmonella. Genus of non-lactose-fermenting, gram-negative rods of the family *Enterobacteriaceae.* *Salmonella* is a common cause of gastrointestinal or septicemic disease in a wide array of animal species, including humans. It is capable of producing a wide range of symptoms in humans, from mild "food poisoning" or gastroenteritis to fatal septicemia. *Salmonella* infection is contracted by ingesting contaminated water, milk, foods that include contaminated uncooked chicken eggs (including ice cream, meringue pies, Hollandaise sauce), and undercooked poultry, beef, pork, and fish. Other foods may be contaminated by infected food handlers or utensils. It is also possible to become infected from handling sick or colonized animals, including turtles and lizards. The taxonomy of this genus has recently undergone drastic revision. It is now proposed that only two species of *Salmonella* are recognized, *S. enterica* and

S. bongori (67). *S. enterica* includes six subspecies, the most important of which is *S. enterica* subsp. *enterica* (also designated as group I). Group I includes most strains commonly isolated from humans and warm-blooded animals, while group II (*S. bongori*) includes those species usually isolated from cold-blooded animals. Embedded in this new nomenclature is another name called the serotype or serovar. There are more than 2,500 different serotypes of the two species (67). Certain of these serotypes represent the well-recognized names of clinically important members of the genus, e.g., typhi, paratyphi, enteritidis, typhimurium, etc. These changes ensure confusion when the literature of the past several decades is reviewed for the clinical and epidemiologic significance of a certain "species" of *Salmonella*. Some of these are reviewed below in an attempt to put the existing literature into perspective along with this new taxonomy. Most clinical microbiology laboratories identify isolates as *Salmonella* species based on biochemical reactivity, and add the cell wall (O-antigen) serogroup designation, e.g., *Salmonella* serogroup B. Public health reference laboratories may be able to further classify important isolates to the serotype level for epidemiologic purposes.

S. arizonae (previously known as *Arizona hinshawii*). Has been isolated from snakes, turtles, fowl, and mammals. In humans, it may produce gastroenteritis, enteric fever, urinary tract infections, bacteremia, meningitis, osteomyelitis, and brain abscess.

S. choleraesuis. May produce a typhoidal type of disease (septicemic) with acute gastroenteritis and enteric fever. Blood-borne dissemination may result in pneumonia, endocarditis, osteomyelitis, abscesses, and meningitis. The natural host is the pig. Some taxonomists argue that *S. choleraesuis* should be the "type species" of *Salmonella*, although the consensus appears to favor *S. enterica* instead.

S. enteritidis. Formerly the most common "species" of *Salmonella*. However, *S. enteritidis* is only a serotype in the new taxonomic nomenclature. It is widely distributed in various animals. In humans, it may produce a gastrointestinal illness or, less commonly, a septicemic typhoidal type of disease. The disease may become disseminated in the septicemic form and may result in abscesses, pneumonia, osteomyelitis, endocarditis, and meningitis.

S. typhi (formerly *S. typhosa*). The serotype that is the causative agent of typhoid fever, which begins as a gastrointestinal infection, but usually presents as a serious septicemic disease that occurs only in humans. Blood cultures are often positive during the first week or two of untreated disease. Stool cultures become positive again after 10 days. A characteristic "rose spots" rash may occur on the trunk in 10 to 15 days. Serious complications include intestinal hemorrhage from ulceration, peritonitis, osteomyelitis, brain abscesses, endo-carditis, meningitis, and abscesses in various organs.

Sarcina. See *Micrococcus* or *Peptostreptococcus.*

Serratia. Genus of gram-negative rods belonging to the family *Enterobacteriaceae.* Most human clinical isolates represent hospital-acquired infections. *Serratia* originally was an organism that produced a bright-red pigment, but most human clinical isolates now lack pigmentation.

S. liquefaciens (formerly *Enterobacter liquefaciens*). Has been isolated occasionally from the respiratory tract, blood, and urinary tract infections. It is the second most frequently isolated species of *Serratia.*

S. marcescens. Widely distributed in nature in soil and water. Once thought to be harmless, red-pigmented strains were used as aerosols to study settling and drifting of bacteria in air currents (98). Now, *S. marcescens* is a fairly common cause of hospital-acquired or dialysis-associated infections. It may produce serious, life-threatening pulmonary infections, empyema, urinary tract infections, otitis externa, eye infections, septicemia, endocarditis, arthritis, chronic osteomyelitis, postoperative wound infections, and meningitis.

S. odorifera. An occasional cause of nosocomial urinary or respiratory tract infections.

S. plymuthica. An occasional cause of nosocomial respiratory tract infections.

S. rubidaea. Has occasionally been isolated from respiratory tract, blood, and wound infections.

Shewanella. Genus of non-glucose-fermenting, gram-negative rods that were formerly named *Pseudomonas putrefaciens*. This genus also includes some even less commonly encountered soil bacteria. Two species are now described, *S. putrefaciens* and *S. alga*. These organisms may cause cellulitis, eye infections, otitis media, abscesses, osteomyelitis, and septicemia associated with an environmental source (18).

Shigella. Genus of pathogenic gram-negative bacilli of the family *Enterobacteriaceae*, most species of which are nonlactose fermenters. It produces bacillary dysentery characterized by blood and mucus in the human large intestine. Infection is almost always limited to the intestine, with rare invasion of the blood stream. Transmission is from human to human by fecal contamination of food or water or by the unwashed hands of food handlers, contaminated utensils, or flies. Historically, *Shigella* has been separated into four serogroups that are treated as species. The treatment of shigellosis is often complicated by multiple antimicrobial resistance of contemporary isolates.

Group A: *S. dysenteriae*. Produces the most severe form of bacillary dysentery, manifests central nervous system symptoms due to production of Shiga toxin, and sometimes results in hemolytic-uremic syndrome (HUS). It is relatively uncommon in the United States, but causes epidemic dysentery in developing countries.

Group B: *S. flexneri*. The second most common species in the United States. Reiter's chronic arthritis syndrome may rarely result from *S. flexneri* infection.

Group C: *S. boydii*. Produces an acute diarrheal disease, most commonly in tropical, developing regions.

Group D: *S. sonnei*. The most commonly isolated species in the United States.

***Sphingobacterium*.** Genus of small, aerobic, gram-negative rods that have been named recently. It is not part of the family *Enterobacteriaceae*, but can be found in soil and water. *S. multivorum* and *S. spiritivorum* are two species that have rarely been associated with peritonitis or bacteremia in humans.

***Sphingomonas*.** A newly named genus of uncommon, aerobic, gram-negative bacilli found in moist areas of the hospital environment, and occasionally as a cause of urinary tract, wound, or bloodstream infections. *S. paucimobilis* (previously *Pseudomonas paucimobilis*) appears to be the most common species.

Spirochetes. A general or group name applied to members of the genus *Treponema* (see below).

***Staphylococcus*.** A very important genus of gram-positive cocci belonging to the family *Micrococcaceae*. Cells are usually arranged in irregular grape-like clusters. Most species represent part of the normal flora of the skin, mucous membranes, and respiratory and gastrointestinal tracts. However, *S. aureus* is recognized as an important pathogen, and some of the coagulase-negative species are often associated with infections of indwelling medical devices (73).

S. aureus. Typically produces an off-white, tan, or golden-yellow colony and produces the enzyme, staphylocoagulase (i.e., is coagulase-positive). This species characteristically produces abscesses in humans and animals. It also causes carbuncles, impetigo, postsurgical wound infections, pneumonia, empyema, osteomyelitis, arthritis, puerperal sepsis, bacteremia, endocarditis, meningitis, brain abscess, scalded-skin syndrome, and "food poisoning" (production of enterotoxins in certain foods). Hospital-acquired strains are often resistant to multiple antibiotics, including methicillin or oxacillin (MRSA strains), and are resistant to several other drug classes. Different MRSA strains have recently become more frequent causes of community-acquired infections, especially skin and soft-tissue infections (41). In recent years, certain *S. aureus* strains (known as VISA or VRSA) have developed either intermediate- or high-level resistance to vancomycin (17, 84). *S. aureus* is a cause of toxic shock syndrome by virtue of producing a systemically absorbed toxin (toxic shock syndrome toxin-1, TSST-1). The latter condition is characterized by fever, sunburn-like rash, and, occasionally, severe hypotension that can lead to death.

S. epidermidis. The most commonly isolated coagulase-negative species. It is generally less virulent than *S. aureus*, producing insidious but potentially very serious infections, such as bacteremia, endocarditis, and infections of catheters and various prosthetic devices. In recent years, multidrug resistance (including methicillin and oxacillin) has become a common feature of this species.

S. intermedius and *S. hyicus.* Two additional coagulase-positive species important in veterinary medicine. While *S. intermedius* is a common pathogen in some animals, it only rarely causes dog-bite infections in humans.

S. saprophyticus. Coagulase-negative species that was once classified as *Micrococcus,* subgroup 3 (43). It has a predilection for the urinary tract, especially in young women, in whom it causes acute cystitis second in frequency to *E. coli.* It rarely causes infections outside the urinary tract.

Other species of coagulase-negative staphylococci. These species, representing normal flora of the skin and mucous membranes, but also causing opportunistic infections in humans similar to those caused by *S. epidermidis,* include *S. haemolyticus, S. hominis, S. warneri, S. lugdunensis, S. simulans, S. schleiferi, S. auricularis* (normally found in the external ear canal), *S. capitis* (human scalp), *S. cohnii, S. caprae, S. pasteuri, S. xylosus,* and *S. saccharolyticus* (an anaerobic species previously named *Peptococcus saccharolyticus)*. Two species deserve further attention, *S. haemolyticus* and *S. lugdunensis*. *S. haemolyticus* is the second most frequently isolated species. It has been associated with bacteremia, endocarditis, and bone and joint infections (52). *S. lugdunensis* has been reported as a frequent cause of native valve endocarditis (88). However, because identification of these organisms to the species level is difficult and the methods are not entirely reliable, many clinical laboratories identify them only as "coagulase-negative staphylococci," with the exception of *S. saprophyticus*. This designation is usually sufficient for clinical purposes, since virtually all the species have the capability of producing very similar device-associated infections (73).

Stenotrophomonas maltophilia. A species of aerobic, non-glucose-fermentative, gram-negative rod that has been reclassified several times in recent years. Formerly known as *Pseudomonas maltophilia*, then *Xanthomonas maltophilia*, it appears to be ubiquitous in soil, water, sewage, and the hospital environment. In humans, it has been incriminated in urinary tract and wound infections, meningitis, septicemia, brain abscesses, peritoneal dialysis-associated infections, conjunctivitis, keratitis, intraocular infections, and various other soft-tissue infections, especially in debilitated individuals (20). It is characterized by multiple antibiotic resistance, making therapy difficult.

Stomatococcus. Genus of gram-positive cocci that represents part of the normal flora of the skin and upper respiratory tract, similar to staphylococci and micrococci. It infrequently causes infection in humans, and is primarily associated with nosocomial infections of medical devices.

Streptobacillus moniliformis. Extremely fastidious, gram-negative, pleomorphic bacillus commonly found in the mouths of wild rats, mice, and cats and transmitted to humans through bites, scratches, or ingestion of milk or water that has been contaminated by rats (Haverhill fever). It is the cause of rat-bite fever, which is characterized by prolonged fever, skin rash, and generalized arthritis (97). It occasionally produces endocarditis and pericarditis.

Streptococcus. Genus of facultative gram-positive cocci from the family *Streptococcaceae* that tend to be arranged in chains of cells. It is widely distributed in nature in water, soil, and vegetation, in milk and other dairy products, and in the respiratory, genitourinary, and gastrointestinal tracts of many animals and humans. Streptococci are capable of producing disease in almost every human organ. Several overlapping, and often confusing and tedious classifications of this genus exist, based on tradition or historical significance, as follows:

Brown classification. Based on the types of hemolysis on animal erythrocytes (usually sheep blood).

Alpha streptococci (viridans group). Characterized by an indistinct zone of partially hemolyzed red blood cells immediately adjacent to colonies and then typically surrounded by green, discolored medium. Included in this category are the streptococci that represent a significant portion of the normal upper respiratory and genitourinary tract flora. *S. pneumoniae* also produces α-hemolysis.

Beta streptococci. Surrounded by a clear, cell-free zone of hemolysis in the agar and include most streptococci of Lancefield groups A, B, C, F, and G.

Gamma streptococci. Produce no change (neither greening nor hemolysis) on blood agar. Types that may be included in this group are *S. bovis* and some of the viridans group streptococci.

Lancefield's classification. Based on antigenic characteristics of group-specific "C" substance in the cell walls of some β-hemolytic streptococci. The groups include:

Group A streptococci. Includes primarily *S. pyogenes*. A β-hemolytic *Streptococcus* that causes erysipelas, scarlet fever, acute glomerulonephritis, rheumatic fever, suppurative infections of the throat, ear, sinuses, mastoids, tonsils; also, peritonsillar abscess, cellulitis, impetigo, lymphadenitis, pneumonia, puerperal sepsis, septicemia, endocarditis, and meningitis. This species is also responsible for streptococcal toxic shock syndrome (81).

Group B streptococci (*S. agalactiae*). β-Hemolytic *Streptococcus* that can be recovered from cervical, vaginal, and rectal cultures of asymptomatic females. It is an important cause of postpartum sepsis, urinary and female genital tract infections, osteomyelitis, septic arthritis, septicemia, endocarditis, meningitis, and especially intrauterine fetal infection (with fulminant fetal or neonatal septicemia, pneumonia, and meningitis). There is an early-onset neonatal disease largely preventable by peripartum antibiotic administration, and a later-onset version that may occur from 1 to 4 weeks after birth

(53). In nonpregnant adults, diabetes, cancer, and HIV infection appear to be predisposing factors to systemic infection (92). It was originally described as a cause of mastitis in cows.

Group C streptococci. β-Hemolytic streptococci that include both large-colony (*S. dysgalactiae* subsp. *equisimilis*) and small-colony versions (*S. anginosus* or *S. milleri* group). They have been isolated from various animals, including horses, cattle, and sheep, and from the respiratory tract of humans. Numerous types of infections in humans include pharyngitis, cellulitis, pneumonia, osteomyelitis, bacteremia, endocarditis, meningitis, and brain abscess.

Group D streptococci. Formerly included the enterococci, which now have their own genus, and nonenterococcal strains, primarily *S. bovis*. This remaining member of the group is a normal inhabitant of the human gastrointestinal tract. Bacteremia caused by *S. bovis* is associated with malignancies of the gastrointestinal tract. It can also cause endocarditis and meningitis.

Group F streptococci. β-Hemolytic streptococci that have been isolated most commonly from the human pharynx. They are also isolated from wounds, abscesses, the genitourinary tract, and blood. These streptococci include members of the *S. anginosus* or *S. milleri* group.

Group G streptococci. β-Hemolytic streptococci that have been isolated from humans and animals. In humans, they have most often been implicated in respiratory tract infections, cellulitis, endocarditis, septicemia, and meningitis. The group includes both large- and small-colony variants, the latter usually belonging to the *S. anginosus* or *S. milleri* group.

Streptococcus **species.** The most modern approach to distinguishing members of this important genus is the establishment of species, based in large part on genetic relatedness. These include the most prominent members of the genus listed below.

S. agalactiae **(group B *Streptococcus*).** Demonstrates predilection for the pregnant female and neonate as described above. It has caused many types of infections in both pregnant and non-pregnant individuals.

S. anginosus. A species group that may also include *S. constellatus* or *S. intermedius*, it is a small-colony group A, C, F, or G β-hemolytic or viridans group *Streptococcus*. It has been isolated from the skin, vagina, and throat. They are designated the *S. milleri* group by British microbiologists, but may be called the species *S. anginosus* by U.S. microbiologists (8). These small-colony hemolytic or nonhemolytic streptococci seem to have a predilection for producing abscesses in various organs and for causing bacteremia.

S. bovis. Perhaps the only remaining member of the Lancefield group D streptococci. *S. bovis* is a cause of bacteremia and endocarditis, and it is occasionally isolated from urine. There is an association between bacteremia caused by this organism and gastrointestinal cancers (51).

S. constellatus. A species clouded in taxonomic history. Formerly referred to as *S. anginosus-constellatus* or *S. MG-intermedius*, this species comprises primarily small-colony group F β-hemolytic or nonhemolytic strains of the *S. milleri* group. It has been isolated from some pulmonary infections.

S. cristatus or *S. crista.* A recently named member of the genus, isolated primarily from dental plaque.

S. dysgalactiae (S. dysgalactiae subsp. equisimilis). A large-colony variant of the β-hemolytic group C or G streptococci. It is an occasional cause of soft-tissue infection or bacteremia in humans.

S. equisimilis. The same as *S. dysgalactiae* subsp. *equisimilis*.

S. faecalis. Now known as *Enterococcus faecalis*. It was formerly a group D enterococcus that may be β-, α-, but most often γ-hemolytic.

S. gordonii. A recently named member of the genus, isolated primarily from dental plaque.

S. intermedius. A species also formerly referred to as *S. anginosus-constellatus* or *S. MG-intermedius*. This species is primarily nonhemolytic, but may have small-colony β-hemolytic strains. It has been isolated primarily from oral infections.

S. milleri. The term emphasized in the United Kingdom to refer to many β-hemolytic and α-hemolytic streptococci, which appear especially able to cause serious suppurative diseases in humans, including abscess formation in many different organs, osteomyelitis, bacteremia, and endocarditis. American taxonomists describe *S. milleri* as a "group" or complex of species to include small-colony β-hemolytic *S. anginosus* (which may possess group A, C, F, or G antigens), as well as *S. intermedius* and *S. constellatus*, which are α- or β-hemolytic (8).

S. mitis. α-Hemolytic and, thus, a member of the viridans group. It is part of the normal upper respiratory tract flora and is found in dental plaque. It has caused bacteremia, endocarditis, and local abscesses. There is also an *S. mitis* "group" that includes *S. mitis, S. sanguis, S. parasanguis, S. gordonii, S. crista, S. oralis, S. peroris,* and *S. infantis.*

S. mutans. A member of the viridans group that has been implicated as a cause of dental caries and, infrequently, a cause of bacterial endocarditis. The *S. mutans* "group" includes *S. mutans, S. sobrinus, S. salivarius, S. bovis*, and *S. vestibularis.*

S. oralis. Has been isolated primarily from dental plaque.

S. pneumoniae (previously *Diplococcus pneumoniae*, pneumococcus). A gram-positive, encapsulated diplococcus. The organism is carried as part of the normal flora of the upper respiratory tract in some individuals, although it is notably the most common cause of bacterial pneumonia, acute sinusitis, otitis media, mastoiditis, and now meningitis in persons more than one month of age. It also is a prominent cause of conjunctivitis, bacteremia, endocarditis, pericarditis, peritonitis, septic arthritis, osteomyelitis, gynecologic infections, and, rarely, urinary tract infections. Penicillin and multiple antibiotic resistance in contemporary pneumococcal isolates (16, 61, 94) often complicates therapy. Two vaccines are now available to protect against invasive pneumococcal infections, one for children, and one for elderly adults or for persons with certain underlying medical conditions that predispose them to invasive pneumococcal disease. The success of the recently released vaccine for children promises to markedly reduce disease in those 2 years of age or younger (93).

S. pyogenes (group A β-hemolytic Streptococcus). A very virulent organism capable of producing innumerable infections in humans. See group A *Streptococcus* description.

S. salivarius. A member of the *S. mutans* group of viridans streptococci. It is part of the normal upper respiratory tract flora. It is an important cause of bacteremia and of endocarditis of dental origin.

S. sanguis. A member of the *S. mitis* group of viridans streptococci. It is found in dental plaque and is one of the most common causes of endocarditis.

S. viridans. Although this is not a legitimate species name and should not be used, it is a common clinical term for α-hemolytic streptococci or for the viridans group of streptococci. Commonly isolated as part of the normal oral and respiratory tract flora, members of this group are capable of producing bacterial endocarditis when heart valves are abnormal. Nutritionally deficient streptococci (vitamin B_6-dependent streptococci, "satelliting" streptococci) were formerly members of this group and are now known as *Abiotrophia* or *Granulacatella* species.

Streptomyces. Aerobic actinomycetes that are usually harmless commensals in soil. However, one species, *S. somaliensis*, causes mycetomas similar to those caused by *Nocardia* species following trauma or contact with soil in tropical areas of the world. These mycetomas are particularly common on the head or neck.

Sutterella. *Sutterella wadsworthensis* is a new name for some strains formerly called *Bacteroides gracilis*. It is an uncommon contributor to anaerobic intra-abdominal infections.

Syphilis. An important sexually transmitted disease caused by *Treponema pallidum* (see below).

Tatumella. A new genus of the family *Enterobacteriaceae* with a single species, *T. ptyseos*. It has occasionally been recovered from clinical specimens, including sputum, urine, and blood.

Treponema. Genus of motile gram-negative spirochetes, some of which are pathogenic, but others are saprophytes. They are best observed under dark-field illumination or by immunofluorescence, because their narrow cell diameter makes visualization difficult with most stains. Diseases caused by the pathogenic treponemas are now referred to as treponematoses. Some new species designations have been promulgated in recent years.

   T. carateum. The etiologic agent of pinta, a nonvenereal skin disease occurring in Mexico, South America, the Philippines, and Pacific areas, primarily in children and adolescents. It is characterized by skin papules, hyperpigmented and depigmented areas, and late involvement of the nervous and cardiovascular systems. It is transmitted by direct skin contact.

***T. pallidum* subsp. *endemicum*.** The spirochete causing "endemic" syphilis or bejel, a nonvenereal disease of children and adults in arid regions of the Middle East and North Africa. It is transmitted by direct mucous membrane contact.

***T. pallidum* subsp. *pallidum*.** The causative spirochete of venereal syphilis, an important sexually transmitted disease with serious multisystem complications. It is distributed worldwide and occurs primarily in adolescents and adults, but it can be a congenital infection. Untreated, the disease can progress from an initial genital lesion (chancre) to secondary and latent stages. Tertiary (late) syphilis usually occurs years after the initial infection, and can result in multiorgan involvement (cardiovascular, skin, bone, central nervous system). Neurosyphilis can occur early or late in infection. Infections in pregnant women can have devastating effects on the fetus, including fetal death or serious developmental problems in the fetus.

T. pallidum subsp. *pertenue.* Causes yaws (frambesia) in tropical countries. The disease is characterized by skin lesions with scars and bone destruction. It occurs primarily in children and is transmitted by direct skin contact.

Tric agent. See *Chlamydia trachomatis.*

Tropheryma. Tropheryma whippelii is the unculturable putative agent of Whipple's disease. It has been visualized microscopically in small-bowel biopsies stained with periodic acid-Schiff (PAS) stain, and can be detected in various tissues by PCR (71). Whipple's disease is a chronic, slowly progressive disease that begins with malabsorption and weight loss, but it may progress to multiorgan involvement that eventually results in a fatal outcome.

Tsukamurella. A genus of aerobic, branching, gram-positive bacilli that occasionally causes infections in immunosuppressed patients. Such infections have included chronic pulmonary, cutaneous, and peritoneal infections, catheter-associated bacteremia, and meningitis. While several species are recognized, infections in humans are most often said to be due to *T. paurometabola.*

Turicella. A genus of aerobic gram-positive bacilli very similar to *Corynebacterium. T. otitidis* has been isolated exclusively from the external ear canal of children, but may not cause otitis media.

TWAR. Now known as *Chlamydophila pneumoniae*.

Typhus. Flea and louse-borne diseases due to various *Rickettsia* species.

Ureaplasma urealyticum. Species of very small gram-negative bacteria that lack a cell wall, formerly classified as T strains of *Mycoplasma*. Present in the genitourinary tracts of virtually all sexually active females and males. Despite their ubiquity in the lower genital tract, there is some evidence to associate *U. urealyticum* with nongonococcal and nonchlamydial urethritis in men and women (83). In addition, there is an association with upper genital tract infections in females, possibly resulting in infertility. These organisms have also been associated with the formation of renal calculi (due to urea splitting). *U. urealyticum* has been recovered from the maternal bloodstream after childbirth or abortion and has been associated with low birth weight and other fetal morbidity in offspring of infected mothers.

Vagococcus. A genus of very uncommon aerobic gram-positive cocci resembling enterococci that has been associated primarily with urinary tract infections.

Veillonella. Genus of anaerobic gram-negative diplococci. *Veillonella* has been isolated from the human respiratory, intestinal, and genitourinary tracts. It is usually considered of low pathogenicity, but *V. parvula* has been associated with other anaerobes in producing various head, neck, and bite-wound infections.

Vibrio. Genus of aerobic, short, slightly curved, motile, gram-negative rods. The natural habitat of *Vibrio* species is generally seawater, brackish water, or occasionally fresh water. They also live in and on various marine animals. Specialized media, including those supplemented with salt, may be required for culture. Infections in humans may result from drinking contaminated water, from ingesting un-cooked or incompletely cooked seafood (especially shellfish), or by skin contact with seawater (especially in association with trauma) (85). A list of some *Vibrio* species that have been isolated from humans follows.

V. alginolyticus. Has been isolated from patients with leg wounds, otitis media, conjunctivitis, and skin infections following exposure to seawater.

V. cholerae (formerly *V. comma*). The etiologic agent of epidemic cholera, an acute and often severe, toxin-mediated diarrheal disease that has caused both epidemics and pandemics (68). Most isolates belong either to serogroup O1 or, more recently, to group O139-Bengal (2). *V. cholerae* has been isolated from contaminated water, fruits, vegetables, and sewage; from inapparent infections; from healthy carriers; and from classic cases of cholera. The greatest complication of clinical cholera is extreme dehydration from massive fluid loss via rice-water stools. Cholera is no longer limited to the Indian subcontinent, but now may be acquired in many temperate regions of the world, including some areas of the Gulf of Mexico.

ic*V. cholerae* non-O1/O139 (formerly noncholera or nonagglutinable vibrios). Closely resemble classical *V. cholerae*, but do not cause epidemic disease. It may cause less severe diarrhea, but also wound infections and fatal bacteremia in patients with chronic liver disease.

ic*V. cincinnatiensis*. A very rare cause of cellulitis, bacteremia, and possibly diarrhea.

ic*V. damselae*. A rare cause of wound infections in humans following contact with the marine environment.

ic*V. fetus*. Now known as *Campylobacter fetus*.

V. fluvialis. Appears to be a cause of sporadic cases of diarrhea, mostly in developing areas of the world.

V. furnissii. A more recently described species that appears to cause diarrhea.

V. hollisae. A recently described *Vibrio* species that appears to cause diarrhea after consumption of raw seafood.

V. jejuni. Now known as *Campylobacter jejuni.*

V. metschnikovii. An extremely rare cause of diarrhea or wound infection following exposure to fresh, brackish, or salt water.

V. mimicus. Has caused diarrhea following consumption of raw seafood, especially oysters, and occasionally wound infections and bacteremia.

V. parahaemolyticus. May contaminate seafood, such as crabs and oysters, and causes a toxin-mediated gastroenteritis if these foods are not properly cooked. It is one of the most common causes of diarrheal illness in Japan.

V. vulnificus. The most virulent of the vibrios and produces aggressive cellulitis following trauma and exposure to seawater (76). A second syndrome consists of rapidly progressive primary bacteremia after consumption of raw seafood (especially oysters) in certain debilitated individuals, such as those with chronic liver disease. Disease due to *V. vulnificus* is often rapidly progressive and fatal in individuals with preexisting liver disease.

VRE. Acronym for vancomycin-resistant enterococci.

Weeksella. A recently described genus of non-glucose-fermentative, gram-negative bacilli. *W. virosa* was previously designated CDC group IIf, and has been isolated principally from genitourinary specimens.

Whipple's disease. See *Tropheryma whippelii.*

Whooping cough. Caused by *Bordetella pertussis.*

Wolinella. Genus of anaerobic gram-negative rods that are associated with periodontitis. Members of this genus are now known as *Campylobacter curvus* and *C. rectus.*

Xanthomonas. Now known as *Stenotrophomonas maltophilia.*

Xenorhabdus. Now known as *Photorhabdus.*

Yersinia. Genus of facultative gram-negative rods of the family *Enterobacteriaceae. Yersinia* was formerly placed in the *Pasteurella* genus.

Y. enterocolitica (formerly *Pasteurella enterocolitica*). Produces ileocecal inflammation and mesenteric lymphadenitis resembling acute appendicitis symptoms (13). Polyarthritis, bacteremia, wound infections, and meningitis have also been reported. *Y. enterocolitica* is usually acquired from ingestion of contaminated water or food in cooler climates. In persons with HLA-B27 histocompatibility antigen, there have been nonsuppurative sequelae, including reactive arthritis, myocarditis, glomerulonephritis, and erythema nodosum due to cross-reactive antibodies formed during infection (86). Because the organism prefers cooler growth temperatures, it has also caused severe transfusion reactions from contaminated blood or blood products kept in blood banks under refrigeration.

Y. pestis (formerly *Pasteurella pestis*). A rodent infection transmitted by fleas, but which humans may acquire. It is the etiologic agent of plague, which, in humans, may occur in three clinical forms: bubonic, septicemic, and primary pneumonic plague. The pneumonic form ("black death") is highly infectious from human to human. In the western United States, the organism may cause sylvatic plague in rodents and may occasionally infect humans through the bite of infected fleas. Lesions may occur in almost all organs by dissemination. Large buboes may form in regional lymph nodes. The organism may be cultured from any of the involved sites, including lymph nodes, blood, sputum, and spinal fluid.

Y. pseudotuberculosis (formerly *Pasteurella pseudotuberculosis*). Primarily an infectious agent of birds, rodents, and other animals and rarely infects humans. However, a Far East scarlet fever-like disease has been described in the former Soviet Republics and Japan. It is characterized by high fever, arthritis, and a scarlet fever-like rash.

Y. frederiksenii, *Y. intermedia*, and *Y. kristensenii*. These, and a few other uncommon species, are environmental organisms that occasionally colonize humans, but appear to be of low pathogenicity in humans.

Yolkenella. Genus of the family *Enterobacteriaceae* that is associated with insects and insect bites, similar to *Photorhabdus*.

Zoonoses. Diseases normally found in animals that may occasionally be transmitted to humans, e.g., anthrax, brucellosis, plague, and tularemia.

Normal microbial flora.

Microorganisms normally residing on body surfaces or in various cavities of the body without invasion or harm to the host are often referred to as "normal flora." The type and numbers vary according to the environments of the surfaces and cavities. These organisms help prevent colonization, invasion, and infection by pathogenic microorganisms. Some of the normal flora in the alimentary tract help synthesize vitamin K, aid in nutrient absorption, and help convert bile pigments and acids in the intestine. Although harmless in their usual sites, normal flora may produce disease if introduced into other areas (especially those body cavities that are normally sterile). Another important related term is "colonization." This implies the presence of a potentially pathogenic organism at one of the sites indicated above, perhaps transiently, but without immediate invasion or disease production. Thus, *Streptococcus pneumoniae* can "colonize" the nasopharynx of healthy individuals, but most microbiologists would not consider it to be "normal flora" of that site.

The following is a compilation of microorganisms that constitute the normal flora encountered in various body sites.

A. Normal flora of mouth and oropharynx
1. Viridans streptococci

2. Coagulase-negative staphylococci
3. *Corynebacterium* spp.
4. *Micrococcus* spp.
5. *Neisseria* spp.
6. *Haemophilus* spp.
7. *Stomatococcus* spp.
8. *Peptostreptococcus* spp.
9. *Fusobacterium* spp.
10. *Porphyromonas* spp.
11. *Prevotella* spp.
12. *Veillonella* spp.
13. *Actinomyces* spp.
14. *Eubacterium* spp.
15. *Bifidobacterium* spp.
16. *Propionibacterium* spp.
17. *Candida* spp.

B. Normal flora of the nose
1. Coagulase-negative staphylococci
2. Viridans streptococci
3. *Neisseria* spp.
4. *Haemophilus* spp.

C. Normal flora of the outer ear
1. Coagulase-negative staphylococci
2. *Corynebacterium* spp.
3. *Propionibacterium* spp.

D. Normal flora of the conjunctivae
   1. Coagulase-negative staphylococci
   2. *Haemophilus* spp.
   3. *Corynebacterium* spp.
   4. *Propionibacterium* spp.
   5. Viridans streptococci

E. Normal flora of the skin
   1. Coagulase-negative staphylococci
   2. *Corynebacterium* spp.
   3. *Staphylococcus aureus*
   4. *Propionibacterium* spp.
   5. Viridans streptococci
   6. *Neisseria* spp.
   7. *Peptostreptococcus* spp.
   8. *Clostridium* spp.
   9. *Candida* spp.

F. Normal flora of the urethra
   1. Coagulase-negative staphylococci
   2. *Corynebacterium* spp.
   3. Viridans streptococci
   4. *Neisseria* spp.
   5. *Bacteroides* spp. and *Fusobacterium* spp.
   6. *Peptostreptococcus* spp.
   7. *Prevotella* and *Porphyromonas*

G. Normal flora of the vagina
   1. *Lactobacillus* spp.

    2. *Peptostreptococcus* spp.
    3. *Corynebacterium* spp.
    4. Viridans streptococci
    5. Staphylococci
    6. *Clostridium* spp.
    7. *Bacteroides* spp.
    8. *Prevotella* and *Porphyromonas*
    9. *Gardnerella vaginalis*
  10. *Candida* spp.

H. Normal flora of the gastrointestinal tract
    1. Small intestine
        a. *Lactobacillus* spp.
        b. *Bacteroides* spp.
        c. *Clostridium* spp.
        d. Enterococci
        e. *Enterobacteriaceae*
        f. Streptococci
    2. Large intestine
        a. *Bacteroides* spp.
        b. *Prevotella* and *Porphyromonas*
        c. *Fusobacterium* spp.
        d. *Clostridium* spp.
        e. *Peptostreptococcus* spp.
        f. *Escherichia coli* and some other *Enterobacteriaceae*
        g. Enterococci
        h. *Lactobacillus* spp.
        i. Streptococci (various)

j. *Acinetobacter* spp.
k. Coagulase-negative staphylococci
l. *Actinomyces* spp.
m. *Bifidobacterium* spp.
n. *Eubacterium* spp.
o. *Candida* spp.

SUGGESTED READINGS

1. Bennet, J. V., and P. S. Brachman (ed.). 1998. *Hospital Infections*, 4th ed. Lippincott-Raven, Philadelphia, Pa.

2. Forbes, B. A., D. F. Sahm, and A. S. Weisfeld (ed.). 2002. *Bailey and Scott's Diagnostic Microbiology*, 11th ed. Mosby-Year Book, St. Louis, Mo.

3. Gilbert, D. N., R. C. Moellering, Jr., and M. A. Sande. 2003. *The Sanford Guide to Antimicrobial Therapy*, 33rd ed. Antimicrobial Therapy, Inc., Hyde Park, Vt.

4. Gorbach, S. L., J. G. Bartlett, and N. R. Blacklow (ed.). 1997. *Infectious Diseases*, 2nd ed. The W.B. Saunders Co., Philadelphia, Pa.

5. Jenson, H. B., and R. S. Baltimore. 2002. *Pediatric Infectious Diseases: Principles and Practices*. The W.B. Saunders Co., Philadelphia, Pa.

6. Koneman, E. W., S. D. Allen, W. J. Janda, P. C. Schreckenberger, and W. C. Winn, Jr. (ed.). 1997. *Color Atlas and Textbook of Diagnostic Microbiology*, 5th ed. Lippincott, Philadelphia, Pa.

7. Mandell, G. L., J. E. Bennett, and R. Dolin (ed.). 2000. *Mandell, Douglas and Bennett's Principles and Practice of*

Infectious Diseases, 5th ed. Churchill Livingstone, New York, N.Y.

8. Murray, P. R., E. J. Baron, J. H. Jorgensen, M. A. Pfaller, and R. H. Yolken (ed.). 2003. *Manual of Clinical Microbiology*, 8th ed. ASM Press, Washington, D.C.

9. Murray, P. R., K. S. Rosenthal, G. S. Kobayashi, and M. A. Pfaller (ed.). 2002. *Medical Microbiology*, 4th ed. Mosby-Year Book, St. Louis, Mo.

10. Schaechter, M., C. Engleberg, B. I. Eisenstein, and G. Medoff (ed.). 1999. *Mechanisms of Microbial Diseases*, 3rd ed. The Williams & Wilkins Co., Baltimore, Md.

REFERENCES

1. **Adachi, R., O. Hammerberg, and H. Richardson.** 1983. Infective endocarditis caused by *Kingella kingae*. *Can. Med. Assoc. J.* **128:**1087–1089.

2. **Albert, M. J.** 1994. *Vibrio cholerae* O139 Bengal. *J. Clin. Microbiol.* **32:**2345–2349.

3. **Altwegg, M., and H. K. Geiss.** 1989. *Aeromonas* as a human pathogen. *Crit. Rev. Microbiol.* **16:**253–286.

4. **Bakken, J. S., J. Krueth, C. Wilson-Nordskog, R. L. Tilden, K. Asanovich, and J. S. Dumler.** 1996. Clinical and laboratory characteristics of human granulocytic ehrlichiosis. *JAMA* **275:**199–205.

5. **Barbour, A. G., and D. Fish.** 1993. The biological and social phenomenon of Lyme disease. *Science* **260:**1610–1616.

6. Bayer, A. S., A. W. Chow, D. Betts, and L. B. Guze. 1978. Lactobacillemia: report of nine cases: important clinical and therapeutic considerations. *Am. J. Med.* **64:**808–813.

7. Bergogne-Berezin, E., and K. J. Towner. 1996. *Acinetobacter* spp. as nosocomial pathogens: microbiological, clinical, and epidemiological features. *Clin. Microbiol. Rev.* **9:**148–165.

8. Bert, F., M. Bariou-Lancelin, and N. Lambert-Zechovsky. 1998. Clinical significance of bacteremia involving the "*Streptococcus milleri*" group: 51 cases and review. *Clin. Infect. Dis.* **27:**385–387.

9. Binford, C. H., W. M. Meyers, and G. P. Walsh. 1982. Leprosy. *JAMA* **247:**2283–2292.

10. Blaser, M. J., J. G. Wells, R. A. Feldman, R. A. Pollard, J. R. Allen, and The Collaborative Diarrheal Disease Study Group. 1983. *Campylobacter* enteritis in the United States: a multicenter study. *Ann. Intern. Med.* **98:**360–365.

11. Bloch, J. C., R. Nadarajah, and R. Jacobs. 1997. *Chryseobacterium meningosepticum*: an emerging pathogen among immunocompromised adults. *Medicine* **76:**30–40.

12. Bodey, G. P., R. Bolivar, V. Fainstein, and L. Jadeja. 1983. Infections caused by *Pseudomonas aeruginosa*. *Rev. Infect. Dis.* **5:**279–313.

13. Bottone, E. J., C. R. Gullans, and M. F. Sierra. 1987. Disease spectrum of *Yersinia enterocolitica* serogroup O:3, the predominant cause of human infection in New York City. *Contrib. Microbiol. Immunol.* **9:**56–90.

14. **Brenner, D. J., D. G. Hollis, G. R. Fanning, and R. E. Weaver.** 1989. *Capnocytophaga canimorsus* sp. nov. (formerly CDC group DF-2), a cause of septicemia following dog bite, and *C. cynodegmi* sp. nov., a cause of localized wound infection following dog bite. *J. Clin. Microbiol.* **27:**231–235.

15. **Burgdorfer, W., A. G. Barbour, S. F. Hayes, J. L. Benach, E. Grunwaldt, and J. P. Davis.** 1982. Lyme disease—a tick-borne spirochetosis? *Science* **216:**1317–1319.

16. **Butler, J. C., J. Hofmann, M. S. Cetron, J. A. Elliott, R. R. Facklam, R. F. Breiman, and the Pneumococcal Sentinel Surveillance Working Group.** 1996. The continued emergence of drug-resistant *Streptococcus pneumoniae* in the United States: an update from the Centers for Disease Control and Prevention's Pneumococcal Sentinel Surveillance System. *J. Infect. Dis.* **174:**986–993.

17. **Centers for Disease Control and Prevention.** 2002. *Staphylococcus aureus* resistant to vancomycin—United States, 2002. *Morb. Mortal. Wkly. Rep.* **51:**565–567.

18. **Chen, Y.-S., Y.-C. Liu, M.-Y. Yen, J. H. Wang, J.-H. Wang, S.-R. Wann, and D.-L. Cheng.** 1997. Skin and soft-tissue manifestations of *Shewanella putrefaciens* infection. *Clin. Infect. Dis.* **25:**225–229.

19. **Das, M., A. D. Bradley, F. R. Cockerill, J. M. Steckelberg, and W. R. Wilson.** 1997. Infective endocarditis caused by HACEK microorganisms. *Annu. Rev. Med.* **48:**25–33.

20. **Denton, M., and K. G. Kerr.** 1998. Microbiological and clinical aspects of infection associated with *Stenotrophomonas maltophilia. Clin. Microbiol. Rev.* **11:**57–80.

21. **Dever, L. L., J. W. Martin, B. Seaworth, and J. H. Jorgensen.** 1992. Varied presentations and responses to therapy of *Mycobacterium haemophilum* infections in patients with AIDS. *Clin. Infect. Dis.* **14:**1195–1200.

22. **Dolan, M. J., M. T. Wong, R. L. Regnery, J. H. Jorgensen, M. Garcia, J. Peters, and D. Drehner.** 1993. Syndrome of *Rochalimaea henselae* adenitis suggesting cat scratch disease. *Ann. Intern. Med.* **118:**331–336.

23. **Donisi, A., M. G. Suardi, S. Casari, M. Longo, G. P. Cadeo, and G. Carosi.** 1996. *Rhodococcus equi* infection in HIV-infected patients. *AIDS* **10:**359–362.

24. **Doran, T. I.** 1999. The role of *Citrobacter* in clinical disease of children: review. *Clin. Infect. Dis.* **28:**384–394.

25. **Drobniewski, F. A.** 1993. *Bacillus cereus* and related species. *Clin. Microbiol. Rev.* **6:**324–338.

26. **Dugan, J. M., S. J. Goldstein, C. E. Chenoweth, C. A. Kauffman, and S. F. Bradley.** 1996. *Achromobacter xylosoxidans* bacteremia: report of four cases and review of the literature. *Clin. Infect. Dis.* **23:**569–576.

27. **Edmond, M. B., J. F. Ober, J. D. Dawson, D. L. Weinbaum, and R. P. Wenzel.** 1996. Vancomycin-resistant enterococcal bacteremia: natural history and atributable mortality. *Clin. Infect. Dis.* **23:**1234–1239.

28. **Edmond, M. B., S. A. Riddler, C. M. Baxter, B. M. Wicklund, and A. W. Pasculle.** 1993. *Agrobacterium*

radiobacter: a recently recognized opportunistic pathogen. *Clin. Infect. Dis.* **16**:388–391.

29. **Faden, H., and D. Dryja.** 1989. Recovery of a unique bacterial organism in human middle ear fluid and its possible role in chronic otitis media. *J. Clin. Microbiol.* **27**:2488–2491.

30. **Falkinham, J. O.** 1996. Epidemiology of infection by non-tuberculous mycobacteria. *Clin. Microbiol. Rev.* **9**:178–215.

31. **Farmer, J. J., III, J. H. Jorgensen, P. A. D. Grimont, R. J. Akhurst, G. O. Poinar, Jr., E. Ageron, G. V. Pierce, J. A. Smith, G. P. Carter, K. L. Wilson, and F. W. Hickman-Brenner.** 1989. *Xenorhabdus luminescens* (DNA hybridization group 5) from human clinical specimens. *J. Clin. Microbiol.* **27**:1594–1600.

32. **Finegold, S. M.** 1995. Overview of clinically important anaerobes. *Clin. Infect. Dis.* **20**:S205–S207.

33. **Fiorino, A. S.** 1996. Intrauterine contraceptive device-associated actinomycotic abscess and actinomyces detection on cervical smear. *Obstet. Gynecol.* **87**:142–149.

34. **Foy, H. M.** 1993. Infections caused by *Mycoplasma pneumoniae* and possible carrier state in different populations of patients. *Clin. Infect. Dis.* **17**(Suppl. 1):37–46.

35. **Frederiksen, W.** 1993. Ecology and significance of *Pasteurellaceae* in man—an update. *Int. J. Med. Microbiol. Virol. Parasitol. Infect. Dis.* **279**:27–34.

36. **Funke, G., A. von Graevenitz, J. E. Claridge III, and K. A. Bernard.** 1997. Clinical microbiology of coryneform bacteria. *Clin. Microbiol. Rev.* **10**:125–159.

37. **Gill, M. V., P. E. Schoch, J. M. Musser, and B. A. Cunha.** 1995. Bacteremia and chorioamnionitis due to cryptic genospecies of *Haemophilus influenzae* biotype I. *Eur. J. Clin. Microbiol. Infect. Dis.* **14**:1088–1090.

38. **Gordon, S., J. S. Swenson, B. C. Hill, N. E. Pigott, R. R. Facklam, R. C. Cooksey, C. Thornsberry, W. R. Jarvis, and F. C. Tenover.** 1992. Antimicrobial susceptibility patterns of common and unusual species of enterococci causing infections in the United States. *J. Clin. Microbiol.* **30**:2373–2378.

39. **Grayson, M. L., W. Tee, and B. Dwyer.** 1989. Gastroenteritis associated with *Campylobacter cinaedi*. *Med. J. Aust.* **150**:214–215.

40. **Greene, K. A., R. J. Clark, and J. M. Zabramski.** 1992. Ventricular CSF shunt infections associated with *Corynebacterium jeikeium*: report of three cases and review. *Clin. Infect. Dis.* **16**:139–141.

41. **Herold, B. C., L. C. Immergluck, M. C. Maranan, D. S. Lauderdale, R. E. Gaskin, S. Boyle-Vavra, C. D. Leitch, and R. S. Daum.** 1998. Community-acquired methicillin-resistant *Staphylococcus aureus* in children with no identifiable predisposing risk. *JAMA* **279**:593–598.

42. **Holst, E., J. Rollof, L. Larsson, and J. P. Nielsen.** 1992. Characterization and distribution of *Pasteurella* species recovered from infected humans. *J. Clin. Microbiol.* **30**:2984–2987.

43. **Hovelius, B., and P.-A. Mardh.** 1984. *Staphylococcus saprophyticus* as a common cause of urinary tract infections. *Rev. Infect. Dis.* **6**:328–337.

44. **Inderlied, C., C. Kempler, and L. Bermudez.** 1993. The *Mycobacterium avium* complex. *Clin. Microbiol. Rev.* **6:**266–310.

45. **Johnson, S., and D. N. Gerding.** 1997. *Clostridium difficile*-associated diarrhea. *Clin. Infect. Dis.* **26:**1027–1036.

46. **Jorgensen, J. H.** 1992. Update on mechanisms and prevalence of antimicrobial resistance in *Haemophilus influenzae. Clin. Infect. Dis.* **14:**1119–1123.

47. **Karulus, R., and A. Campagnari.** 2000. *Moraxella catarrhalis*: a review of an important human mucosal pathogen. *Microbes Infect.* **2:**547–559.

48. **Kawamura, Y., X. Hou, F. Sultana, S. Liu, H. Yamamoto, and T. Ezaki.** 1995. Transfer of *Streptococcus adjacens* and *Streptococcus defectivus* to *Abiotrophia* gen. nov. as *Abiotrophia adiacens* comb. nov. and *Abiotrophia defectiva* comb. nov., respectively. *Int. J. Syst. Bacteriol.* **45:**798–803.

49. **Kaye, J. M., A. Macone, and P. H. Kazanjian.** 1992. Catheter infection caused by *Methylobacterium* in immunocompromised hosts: report of three cases and review of the literature. *Clin. Infect. Dis.* **14:**1010–1014.

50. **Kirchner, J. T.** 1991. *Clostridium septicum* infection. Beware of associated cancer. *Postgrad. Med.* **90:**157–160.

51. **Klein, R. S., M. T. Catalano, S. C. Edberg, J. I. Casey, and N. H. Steigbigel.** 1979. *Streptococcus bovis* septicemia and carcinoma of the colon. *Ann. Intern. Med.* **91:**560–562.

52. **Kloos, W. E., and T. L. Bannerman.** 1994. Update on clinical significance of coagulase-negative staphylococci. *Clin. Microbiol. Rev.* **7:**117–140.

53. **Krohn, M. A., S. L. Hillier, and C. J. Baker.** 1999. Maternal peripartum complications associated with vaginal Group B streptococci colonization. *J. Infect. Dis.* **179:**1410–1415.

54. **Leelarasmee, A., and S. Bovornkitti.** 1989. Meliodosis: review and update. *Rev. Infect. Dis.* **11:**413–425.

55. **Lerner, P. I.** 1996. Nocardiosis. *Clin. Infect. Dis.* **22:**891–905.

56. **Lin, F.-Y. C., W. F. Devoe, C. Morrison, J. Libonati, P. Powers, R. J. Gross, B. Rowe, E. Israel, and J. G. Morris.** 1987. Outbreak of neonatal *Citrobacter diversus* meningitis in a suburban hospital. *Pediatr. Infect. Dis. J.* **6:**50–55.

57. **LiPuma, J. J.** 1998. *Burholderia cepacia*: management issues and new insights. *Clin. Chest Med.* **19:**473–486.

58. **Lorber, B.** 1997. Listeriosis. *Clin. Infect. Dis.* **24:**1–11.

59. **Mackenzie, A., L. A. Fuite, F. T. H. Chan, J. King, U. Allen, N. MacDonald, and F. Diaz-Mitoma.** 1995. Incidence and pathogenicity of *Arcanobacterium haemolyticum* during a 2-year study in Ottawa. *Clin. Infect. Dis.* **21:**177–181.

60. **Marshall, B. J.** 1994. *Helicobacter pylori. Am. J. Gastroenterol.* **89:**S116–S128.

61. **McCracken, G. H., Jr.** 1995. Emergence of resistant *Streptococcus pneumoniae*: a problem in pediatrics. *Pediatr. Infect. Dis. J.* **14:**424–428.

62. **McNeil, M. M., and J. M. Brown.** 1994. The medically important aerobic actinomycetes: epidemiology and microbiology. *Clin. Microbiol. Rev.* **7:**357–417.

63. **McQuiston, J. H., C. D. Paddock, R. C. Holman, and J. E. Childs.** 1999. The human ehrlichiosis in the United States. *Emerg. Infect. Dis.* **5:**635–642.

64. **Michaels, R. H., and O. Ali.** 1993. A decline in *Haemophilus influezae* type b meningitis. *J. Pediatr.* **122:**407–409.

65. **Murray, B. E.** 2000. Vancomycin-resistant enterococcal infections. *N. Engl. J. Med.* **342:**710–721.

66. **Pers, C., B. Gahrn-Hansen, and W. Frederiksen.** 1996. *Capnocytophaga canimorsus* septicemia in Denmark, 1982–1985: review of 39 cases. *Clin. Infect. Dis.* **23:**71–75.

67. **Popoff, M. Y., J. Bockemühl, and F. W. Hickman-Brenner.** 1997. Supplement 1996 (no. 40) to the Kauffmann-White schema. *Res. Microbiol.* **148:**811–814.

68. **Raufman, J.-P.** 1997. Cholera. *Am. J. Med.* **104:**386–394.

69. **Raoult, D., H. Tissot-Dupont, C. Foucault, J. Gouvernet, P. E. Fournier, E. Bernit, A. Stein, M. Nesri, J. R. Harle, and P. J. Weiler.** 2000. Q fever 1985–1998, clinical and epidemiological features of 1383 infections. *Medicine (Baltimore)* **79:**109–123.

70. **Reiner, S. L., J. M. Harrelson, S. E. Miller, G. B. Hill, and H. A. Gallis.** 1987. Primary actinomycosis of an extremity: a case report and review. *Rev. Infect. Dis.* **9:**581–589.

71. **Relman, D. A., T. M. Schmidt, R. P. McDermott, and S. Falkow.** 1992. Identification of uncultured bacillus of Whipple's disease. *N. Engl. J. Med.* **327:**293–301.

72. **Rice, L. B.** 2001. Emergence of vancomycin-resistant enterococci. *Emerg. Infect. Dis.* **7:**183–187.

73. **Rupp, M. E., and G. L. Archer.** 1994. Coagulase-negative staphylococci: pathogens associated with medical progress. *Clin. Infect. Dis.* **19:**231–245.

74. **Scott, M. A., T. L. McCurley, C. L. Vnencakjones, C. Hager, J. A. McCoy, B. Anderson, R. D. Collins, and K. M. Edward.** 1996. Cat scratch disease—detection of *Bartonella henselae* DNA in archival biopsies from patients with clinically, serologically, and histologically defined disease. *Am. J. Pathol.* **149:**2161–2167.

75. **Shandera, W. X., C. O. Tacket, and P. A. Blake.** 1983. Food poisoning due to *Clostridium perfringens* in the United States. *J. Infect. Dis.* **147:**167–170.

76. **Shapiro, R. L., S. Altekruse, L. Hutwagner, R. Bishop, R. Hammond, S. Wilson, B. Ray, S. Thompson, R. V. Tauxe, P. M. Griffin, and the *Vibrio* Working Group.** 1998. The role of gulf coast oysters harvested in warmer months in *Vibrio vulnificus* infections in the United States, 1988–1996. *J. Infect. Dis.* **178:**752–759.

77. **Sriram, S., C. W. Stratton, Y. Song-Yi, A. Tarp, L. Ding, J. D. Bannan, and W. M. Mitchel.** 1999. *Chlamydia pneumoniae* infection of the central nervous system in multiple sclerosis. *Ann. Neurol.* **46:**6–14.

78. **Slater, L. N., J. Guarnaccia, S. Makintubee, and G. R. Istre.** 1990. Bacteremic disease due to *Haemophilus*

influenzae capsular type f in adults: report of five cases and review. *Rev. Infect. Dis.* **12**:628–635.

79. **Slutsker, L., A. A. Ries, K. Maloney, J. G. Wells, K. D. Greene, P. M. Griffin, and the *Escherichia coli* O157:H7 Study Group.** 1997. A nationwide case-control study of *Escherichia coli* O157:H7 infection in the United States. *J. Infect. Dis.* **177**:962–966.

80. **Steere, A. C., R. L. Grodzicki, A. N. Kornblatt, J. E. Craft, A. G. Barbour, W. Burgdorfer, G. P. Schmid, E. Johnson, and S. E. Malawista.** 1983. The spirochetal etiology of Lyme disease. *N. Engl. J. Med.* **308**:733–742.

81. **Stevens, D. L.** 1995. Streptococcal toxic-shock syndrome: spectrum of disease, pathogenesis, and new concepts in treatment. *Emerg. Infect. Dis.* **3**:69–78.

82. **Struthers, M., J. Wong, and J. M. Janda.** 1996. An initial appraisal of the clinical significance of *Roseomonas* species associated with human infections. *Clin. Infect. Dis.* **23**:729–733.

83. **Taylor-Robinson, D.** 1996. Infections due to species of *Mycoplasma* and *Ureaplasma*: an update. *Clin. Infect. Dis.* **23**:671–684.

84. **Tenover, F. C., M. V. Lancaster, B. C. Hill, C. D. Steward, S. A. Stocker, G. A. Hancock, C. M. O'Hara, N. C. Clark, and K. Hiramatsu.** 1998. Characterization of staphylococci with reduced susceptibilities to vancomycin and other glycopeptides. *J. Clin. Microbiol.* **36**:1020–1027.

85. **Tison, D. L., and M. T. Kelly.** 1984. *Vibrio* species of medical importance. *Diagn. Microbiol. Infect. Dis.* **2**:263–276.

86. **Toivanen, P., and A. Toivanen.** 1994. Does *Yersinia* induce autoimmunity? *Int. Arch. Allergy Immunol.* **104**:107–111.

87. **Uttamchandani, R. B., G. L. Daikos, R. R. Reyes, M. A. Fischl, G. M. Dickinson, E. Yamaguchi, and M. R. Kramer.** 1994. Nocardiosis in 30 patients with advanced human immunodeficiency virus infection: clinical features and outcome. *Clin. Infect. Dis.* **18**:348–353.

88. **Vandenesch, F., J. Etienne, M. E. Reverdy, and S. J. Eykyn.** 1993. Endocarditis due to *Staphylococcus lugdunensis*: report of 11 cases and review. *Clin. Infect. Dis.* **17**:871–876.

89. **Vickers, R. M., V. L. Yu, S. S. Hanna, P. Muraca, W. Diven, N. Carmen, and F. B. Taylor.** 1987. Determinants of *Legionella pneumophila* contamination of water systems; 15 hospital prospective study. *Infect. Control* **8**:357–363.

90. **Wallace, R. J., Jr., J. M. Swenson, V. A. Silcox, R. C. Good, J. A. Tschen, and M. S. Stone.** 1983. Spectrum of disease due to rapidly growing mycobacteria. *Rev. Infect. Dis.* **5**:657–679.

91. **Wallace, R. J., Jr., M. Tsukamura, B. A. Brown, J. Brown, V. A. Steingrube, Y. S. Zhang, and W. R. Jarvis.** 1990. Cefotaxime-resistant *Nocardia asteroides* strains are isolates of the controversial species *Nocardia farcinica*. *J. Clin. Microbiol.* **28**:2726–2732.

92. **Wessels, M. R., and D. L. Kasper.** 1993. The changing spectrum of group B streptococcal disease. *N. Engl. J. Med.* **328:**1843–1844.

93. **Whitney, C. G., M. F. Farley, J. Hadler, L. H. Harrison, N. M. Bennett, R. Lynfield, A. Reingold, P. R. Cieslak, T. Pilishvili, D. Jackson, R. R. Facklam, J. Jorgensen, and A. Schuchat.** 2003. Decline in invasive pneumococcal disease following the introduction of protein-polysaccharide conjugate vaccine. *N. Engl. J. Med.* **348:**1737–1746.

94. **Whitney, C. G., M. M. Farley, J. Hadler, L. H. Harrison, C. Lexau, A. Reingold, L. Lefkowitz, P. R. Cieslak, M. Cetron, E. R. Zell, J. H. Jorgensen, and A. Schuchat.** 2000. Increasing prevalence of multidrug-resistant *Streptococcus pneumoniae* in the United States. *N. Engl. J. Med.* **343:**1917–1924.

95. **Wong, Y. K., K. D. Dawkins, and M. E. Ward.** 1999. Circulating *Chlamydia pneumoniae* DNA as a predictor of coronary artery disease. *J. Am. Coll. Cardiol.* **34:**1435–1439.

96. **Wood, R. C., K. L. MacDonald, and M. T. Osterholm.** 1992. *Campylobacter* enteritis outbreaks associated with drinking raw milk during youth activities. A 10-year review of outbreaks in the United States. *JAMA* **268:**3228–3230.

97. **Wullenweber, M.** 1994. *Streptobacillus moniliformis*—a zoonotic pathogen. Taxonomic considerations, host species, diagnosis, therapy, geographical distribution. *Lab. Anim.* **29:**1–15.

98. **Yu, V. L.** 1979. *Serratia marcescens*: historical perspective and clinical review. *N. Engl. J. Med.* **300:**887–893.

Fungi

Absidia corymbifera. A member of the class *Zygomycetes* in the order *Mucorales*, *A. corymbifera* is a filamentous fungus (mold) characterized by broad sparsely septate, hyaline hyphae with stolons and internodal rhizoids. As with other members of the *Zygomycetes*, this species has a worldwide distribution in soil and decaying vegetation. *A. corymbifera* is a rare agent of zygomycosis, causing invasive infections in immunocompromised individuals (e.g., patients with neutropenia, AIDS, or metabolic acidosis). Treatment options include amphotericin B, usually accompanied by surgical excision of the infected tissue (5,14).

Acremonium. Formerly known as *Cephalosporium*, this ubiquitous mold is found in soil and decaying plant material. *Acremonium* manifests septate hyaline hyphae and produces one-celled conidia in slimy masses or chains at the tips of the phialides. It may be confused with *Fusarium* species in culture or in tissue. *Acremonium* is an etiologic agent of mycetomas, onychomycosis, keratitis, endocarditis, and meningitis. Several species exist, but species-level identification is difficult and not usually performed. It is variably susceptible to amphotericin B, flucytosine, and azole antifungal agents.

Aleurioconidia. An older term describing conidia (spores) that typically have broad bases of attachment to conidiogenous cells and separate by lysis of conidiogenous hyphal walls, leaving remnants attached to the conidium as an annular frill.

Alternaria. *Alternaria* is a dematiaceous (olive, brown, gray, or black pigmented) mold found on plants, in the soil, and on various foodstuffs. The most common species is *A. alternata*. The hyphae are septate with brown pigmentation. Conidia are irregular in shape, brown, and formed in long branching chains. *Alternaria* is a frequent cause of sinusitis and may also cause keratitis, onychomycosis, subcutaneous phaeohyphomycosis, and, rarely, more widespread invasive infections. In addition to surgical intervention, treatment options include amphotericin B and the azole antifungals.

Anamorph. The asexual form of conidiogenous fungus.

Angioinvasive. The tendency of certain fungi (e.g., *Aspergillus, Pseudallescheria boydii, Zygomycetes*) to invade blood vessels, blocking the lumen of the vessel and causing death of the tissue deprived of blood supply (infarction).

Anthropophilic. Preference of certain dermatophytic fungi to infect humans; animals are rarely infected by these species (e.g., *Epidermophyton floccosum, Microsporum audouini,* and *Trichophyton rubrum*).

Apophysomyces elegans. A member of the class *Zygomycetes* in the order *Mucorales*. It is a mold and forms broad, hyaline, sparsely septate hyphae with foot cells and rhizoids that occur beneath or to the side of sporangiophores. *A. elegans* is an agent of zygomycosis marked by angioinvasion with subsequent necrotizing fasciitis. Infections often occur following traumatic implantation (accidental injury, surgery, burns) in otherwise immunocompetent individuals. Therapy includes aggressive surgical resection of infected tissue plus administration of amphotericin B (5,14).

Arthroconidium. An asexual propagule (spore) formed by the breaking up of a hypha at the point of septation, resulting in a rectangular or barrel-shaped spore.

Ascospore. Asexual spore produced in a sac-like structure known as an *ascus*.

Aspergillus. A genus of hyaline molds that are ubiquitous in nature and found in soil, air, and decaying vegetation. Numerous species of *Aspergillus* have been described as opportunistic pathogens. *A. fumigatus* is the most common species. Other species of clinical importance include *A. flavus, A. versicolor, A. niger, A. glaucus,* and *A. terreus.* Hyphae are hyaline and septate; they often (but not always) branch at 45° angles in tissue. The spectrum of disease includes airway colonization, external otitis, allergy, sinusitis, aspergilloma, invasive pulmonary disease, invasion of the central nervous system, and disseminated infection. The organism is angioinvasive and most commonly infects individuals who are neutropenic or otherwise immunocompromised. Therapeutic options include amphotericin B, caspofungin (an echinocandin), voriconazole, or itraconazole. When possible, immune reconstitution and/or surgical intervention are effective adjuncts to antifungal therapy. Notably, *A. terreus* is considered to be routinely resistant to amphotericin B (8,10).

Aureobasidium pullulans. An opportunistic mold found on plants and in moist environments. *A. pullulans* manifests both hyaline septate hyphae and dematiaceous hyphae, which differentiate to form thick, darkly pigmented arthroconidia. Hyaline blastoconidia may also be produced from hyaline hyphae. *A. pullulans* has been described as the etiologic agent of keratitis and peritonitis, and as an agent of phaeohyphomycosis. It may also represent an insignificant "contaminant" when recovered from cutaneous sites on humans. This organism is generally susceptible to amphotericin B, flucytosine and the azole antifungal agents.

Ballistoconidium. A single-celled spore that is forcibly discharged from a sporophore by hydrostatic pressure. See *Basidiobolus ranarum* and *Conidiobolus coronatus*.

Basidiobolus ranarum. A member of the class *Zygomycetes* in the order *Entomophthorales*, this mold is characterized by broad, sparsely septate hyphae and thick-walled intercalary "beaked" zygospores. Sporangiophores may be "swollen" and forcibly discharge spores, or they may be elongate and passively release spores. The organisms may be isolated from soil and decaying plants, as well as from reptiles and amphibians. *B. ranarum* causes subcutaneous zygomycosis involving the trunk and extremities and presenting as large, firm, nonulcerating cutaneous masses. This organism rarely may invade blood vessels and cause infections resembling those caused by members of the order *Mucorales* (*Absidia, Rhizopus, Mucor*). Subcutaneous zygomycosis is variably responsive to antifungal therapy, including amphotericin B, keto-conazole, itraconazole, trimethoprim/sulfamethoxa-zole, and potassium iodide.

Beauveria. A hyaline mold with septate hyphae, *Beauveria* is found in soil and is known to be pathogenic in some animals and insects. It rarely produces infection in humans, but it has been reported to cause keratitis and pulmonary infections.

Bipolaris. A dematiaceous mold found in soil, air, and vegetation, *Bipolaris* has hyphae that are septate, brown, with zigzag (geniculate) conidiophores bear-ing oblong, thick-walled, brown conidia with three to five septations. Species include *B. australiensis,* *B. cynodontis, B. hawaiiensis,* and *B. spicifera.* Infections include sinusitis, endocarditis, keratitis, endophthalmitis, and pulmonary and central nervous system infections. *B. spicifera* is the most common species causing disease in humans. *B. hawaiiensis* is especially aggressive with a predilection for the central nervous system, and should be handled with care in the laboratory. Most species of *Biopolaris* are sus-ceptible to amphotericin B and the azoles (1).

Blastomyces dermatitidis. A thermally dimorphic pathogen, *B. dermatitidis* grows as a hyaline, septate mold with round or pear-shaped conidia at 25°C and as a large, thick-walled, broad-based, budding yeast at 37°C in culture and in tissue. The organism inhabits soil and is geographically delimited to the Ohio-Mississippi River Valley region. Infections may be asymptomatic or manifest as pulmonary, cutaneous, osteoarticular, or genitourinary tract disease. Disease in both humans and animals is seen in endemic areas. Cultures for *B. dermatitidis* should be handled in a biological safety cabinet to minimize the risk of infection due to inhalation of aerosols. Recommended treatment for blastomycosis is amphotericin B or itraconazole (less serious infections).

Candida. The most common cause of invasive mycosis. Members of the genus *Candida* are small budding yeasts, most of which are capable of forming pseudohyphae and true septate hyphae in culture and in tissue. Most *Candida* species are found as colonizers of human skin and mucosal surfaces and may cause infections ranging from superficial cutaneous and mucosal infections to candidemia and hematogenously disseminated infections. Hematogenous dissemination may result in renal, hepatic, and splenic abscesses, endophthalmitis, osteomyelitis, or meningitis. More than 17 species of *Candida* have been implicated in diseases in humans but the most common causes of infection are *C. albicans, C. glabrata, C. parapsilosis, C. tropicalis, C. krusei,* and *C. lusitaniae.* Therapeutic options for most species include amphotericin B, fluconazole, flucytosine, itraconazole, voriconazole, and caspofungin. When possible, removal of catheters, shunts, and other implanted devices is recommended in patients with hematogenous disease. *C. parapsilosis*, in particular, is known to cause catheter-associated candidemia. *C. glabrata* is less susceptible to fluconazole than other species, requiring higher doses (800 mg/day) for optimal treatment. Approximately 10% of *C. glabrata* isolates are resistant to fluconazole (minimal inhibitory concentration [MIC], ≥ 64 µg/ml) and will also exhibit resistance to voriconazole and itraconazole, but not to caspofungin. *C. krusei* is innately resistant to fluconazole and flucytosine, but it remains susceptible to both voriconazole and caspofungin. Both *C. glabrata* and *C. krusei* are less susceptible to amphotericin B than other species of *Candida* and may require high doses (1 mg/kg/day) for optimal treatment. *C. lusitaniae* may develop secondary resistance to amphotericin B during the course of therapy (1,4,6).

Chaetomium. *Chaetomium* is a dematiaceous mold of the phylum *Ascomycota*. It is characterized by hyaline septate hyphae with dark-pigmented (olive, brown, or gray), round, oval, or flask-shaped perithecia, which contain asci and ascospores. *Chaetomium* is an environmental mold found in soil, air, and decaying vegetation. Infections caused by *Chaetomium* are rare but include onychomycosis, cutaneous lesions, peritonitis, and more widely disseminated infection in immunocompromised individuals. *C. strumarium* is reported to cause fatal brain abscesses in i.v. drug users and may have neurotropic potential.

Chitin. Important structural carbohydrate component of fungal cell wall.

Chlamydoconidium. An enlarged, rounded conidium (spore) that is thick walled and contains stored food. It may be present singly or in chains at the end of the hypha (terminal) or inserted along the hypha (intercalary).

Chromoblastomycosis. Chromoblastomycosis describes a chronic infection of subcutaneous tissues caused by dematiaceous fungi, including *Cladophia-lophora carrionii, Fonsecaea pedrosoi,* and *Phialo-phora verrucosa.* Lesions are usually on the lower extremities and contain planate-dividing, copper-colored, yeast-like bodies also known as sclerotic bodies, Medlar bodies, or muriform cells. Chromo-blastomycosis is usually restricted to tropical and subtropical areas (1,11,12).

Chrysosporium. A hyaline mold characterized by septate hyphae and both single-celled aleurioconidia and chains of alternating arthroconidia; it may be confused with the mold phase of *Blastomyces dermatitidis* in culture. *Chrysosporium* is found commonly in soil and plant material. It is a rare cause of onychomycosis and cutaneous infections.

Cladophialophora. These dematiaceous molds are characterized by pigmented, septate hyphae with long chains of conidia. Species include *C. bantiana,* *C. boppii,* and *C. carrionii*, all of which are widely distributed in soil and plant debris. These species may cause both phaeohyphomycosis and chromoblastomycosis. Importantly, *C. bantiana* appears to be neurotropic and causes phaeophyphomycotic brain abscesses in both immune-competent and immunocompromised hosts. It should be handled with care in a biological safety cabinet. Treatment options include surgery plus itraconazole or fluconazole. Susceptibility to flucytosine and amphotericin B has also been reported.

Cladosporium. These dematiaceous molds, found in air and dead organic matter, are characterized by dark septate hyphae with branching chains of conidia. *Cladosporium* species may cause cutaneous and ocular (keratitis) infections and rarely pulmonary, sinus, or disseminated infections. They are also commonly isolated from foods stored at refrigerator or ambient temperatures.

Clamp connection. A specialized structure forming a bridge over a hyphal septum in the *Basidiomycetes*.

Cleistothecium. A large, rounded, many-celled structure in which asci and ascospores are formed and held until the structure bursts.

Coccidioides immitis. This endemic dimorphic pathogen is localized to the southwestern United States, Northern Mexico, and areas in Central and South America. *C. immitis* grows as a hyaline mold and produces unicellular, barrel-shaped arthroconidia, which alternate with empty disjunctor cells. The arthroconidia are produced in culture and in nature and are highly infectious. In tissue, the organism forms large spherules containing multiple endospores. Infection takes place by inhalation and may be asymptomatic or present as a self-limited pulmonary process, chronic pneumonia, or disseminated disease. Dissemination may produce cutaneous lesions, osteomyelitis, and/or meningitis. Treatment options include fluconazole, itraconazole, or amphotericin B. Cultures must be handled with great care in a biological safety cabinet because of the highly infectious arthroconidia.

Coenocytic. Sparsely septate hyphal structures containing more than one nucleus within an individual cell. Characteristic of *Zygomycetes*.

Cokeromyces recurvatis. A member of the class *Zygomycetes* in the order *Mucorales*, *C. recurvatis* is a mold characterized by broad, hyaline, sparsely septate hyphae, sporangiophores bearing recurving sporangiole stalks, and the development of zygospores in culture. The organism is also capable of forming large (30 to 90 μm) thin-walled yeast cells at 35 to 37°C in 5 to 7% CO_2 with multipolar budding, which may mimic the "mariner's wheel" seen with *Paracoccidiodes brasiliensis*. *C. recurvatis* may be recovered from soil and the droppings of various animals. This organism has been recovered from genitourinary specimens (bladder, vagina, endocervix), pleural and peritoneal fluids, but tissue invasion has not been documented. The role of *C. recurvatis* as an etiologic agent of invasive mycosis has not been established.

Conidiobolus coronatus. A member of the class *Zygomycetes* in the order *Entomophthorales*, this mold is characterized by broad, sparsely septate hyphae. Spores are forcibly discharged from unbranched sporangiophores and may cover the lid and sides of the culture tube or plate. The organism may be isolated from soil, decaying matter, and insects in tropical areas. Conidiobolomycosis is endemic in Central and South America, Southeast Asia, and Africa. The route of infection is by direct inoculation via minor trauma or insect bites. *C. coronatus* causes a chronic granulomatous inflammation involving the nasal mucosa and adjacent subcutaneous tissue. The disease can be quite disfiguring and is characterized by subcutaneous masses and gross facial swelling. In tissue, the organism demonstrates broad ribbon-like, sparsely septate hyphae. The Splendore-Hoeppli phenomenon, characterized by eosinophilic deposits surrounding hyphal elements, may also be seen on histopathologic examination of infected tissues. Angioinvasion, more typical of the *Mucorales*, is rarely seen with *C. coronatus* infections. Treatment includes surgical resection with or without administration of potassium iodide, ketoconazole, amphotericin B, itraconazole, co-trimoxazole, trimethoprim/sulfamethoxazole, fluconazole, or terbinafine, alone or in combination.

Conidiogeneous cell. The cell that produces the conidia.

Conidiophore. A specialized hyphal structure that serves as a stalk on which conidia are formed.

Conidium. Asexual spores that are borne naked (not enclosed in a sac-like structure) at the end of a specialized structure or conidiophore.

Cryptococcus. Encapsulated budding yeasts that are urease-positive and have a worldwide distribution,

Cryptococcus may be isolated from humans and other mammals, soil, fruit, leaves, and pigeon droppings. Numerous species exist, including *C. neoformans, C. albidus, C. laurentii,* and *C. uniguttulatus.* Only *C. neoformans* is considered pathogenic; however, other species have also been isolated from cerebrospinal fluid (CSF), blood, sputum, and peritoneal fluid. There are two varieties of *C. neoformans,* var. *neoformans* and var. *gatti. C. neoformans* var. *neoformans* is found worldwide, is often associated with pigeon droppings, and is a major cause of meningitis in immunocompromised individuals (especially HIV-infected). It may also cause meningitis in nonimmunocompromised individuals. Other clinical manifestations include pulmonary, cutaneous, and disseminated infections. *C. neoformans* var. *gatti* may cause a similar spectrum of disease but is largely restricted to tropical and subtropical regions and has an epidemiologic association with eucalyptus trees. Treatment options include amphotericin B with or without flucytosine and fluconazole (maintenance therapy).

Cunninghamella. A genus in the class *Zygomycetes* in the order *Mucorales,* this mold has a worldwide distribution in decaying matter and soil and may be recovered from cheese. The most common species is *C. bertholletiae,* which is characterized by the presence of broad, sparsely septate hyphae, rhizoids, and sporangiophores ending in large swollen vesicles covered with spine-like denticles, each supporting a sporangium. *Cunninghamella* is an infrequent cause of invasive zygomycosis, including pneumonia and disseminated disease. Treatment includes amphotericin B supplemented by surgical resection of the involved tissue (5,14).

Curvularia. A dematiaceous mold with worldwide distribution as a plant pathogen, *Curvularia* is characterized by dark septate hyphae, bent, knobby conidiophores, and large, curved conidia containing four cells. It is an agent of phaeohyphomycosis involving various sites, including sinus, subcutaneous, ocular (keratitis), pulmonary, and disseminated disease. Surgery plus administration of itraconazole or amphotericin B is the recommended treatment.

Dematiaceous. Having structures containing a melanotic pigment, hyphae, and/or spores that are brown or black.

Denticle. Short, narrow projection bearing a conidium.

Dermatophyte. A fungus belonging to the genus *Trichophyton, Epidermophyton,* or *Microsporum.* These fungi have the ability to infect skin, hair, or nails of humans or animals.

Disjunctor cell. Empty, thin-walled cells separating arthroconidia of *Coccidioides immitis*. As the walls of the disjunctor cells deteriorate, the arthroconidia become detached and disperse.

Drechslera. A dematiaceous mold found on vegetation, this organism produces dark-brown septate hyphae with poor conidiation. Conidia are large and multicelled; they germinate at right angles to the conidial axis. This organism has not been described as an etiologic agent of phaeohyphomycosis. Earlier reports of disease attributed to *Drechslera* were actually caused by another dematiaceous fungus, *Bipolaris*.

Epidermophyton. A dermatophytic mold of worldwide distribution. *Epidermophyton* is characterized by hyaline septate hyphae and large, club-shaped, septate macroconidia. No microconidia are produced. This organism is anthropophilic and is easily spread from person to person. It causes cutaneous infections involving feet (tinea pedis) and groin (tinea cruris). Treatment options include a variety of topical agents and oral terbinafine, ketoconazole, fluconazole, or griseofulvin (3).

Exerohilum. A dematiaceous mold found on plants and grasses and in the soil. *Exerohilum* is characterized by dark septate hyphae and long, thick-walled conidia with 7 to 11 septa. The most common species is *E. rostratum*. *Exerohilum* causes sinusitis and subcutaneous and deep phaeohyphomycosis. Surgery plus administration of itraconazole or amphotericin B is the treatment of choice.

Exophiala. This dematiaceous mold, found in decaying wood, soil, and water, produces hyphae that are olivaceous black, septate, with numerous conidiogenous cells. Conidia gather in clusters at the ends and sides of conidiophores. *Exophiala* may also grow in culture as a black budding yeast. *Exophiala* species may cause subcutaneous and disseminated phaeohyphomycosis, mycetoma, and chromoblastomycosis. Treatment includes surgical resection plus administration of itraconazole or amphotericin B.

Fonsecaea. Found in rotten wood and soil, *Fonsecaea* is characterized by dark septate hyphae that are branched. Conidia formation is complex with conidia borne singly or in chains with or without branching. *F. pedrosoi* is the most common species, but both *F. pedrosoi* and *F. compacta* are agents of chromoblastomycosis in tropical and subtropical areas. Antifungal therapy includes itraconazole (recommended), fluconazole, or terbinafine. Surgical resection is also recommended.

Fusarium. A hyaline mold with broad distribution in soil and on plants, *Fusarium* species are destructive plant pathogens and most are capable of producing mycotoxins that may be detrimental to humans if ingested. *Fusarium* is characterized by septate, branching hyphae with sickle-shaped macroconidia and usually abundant microconidia. In tissue *Fusarium* may resemble *Aspergillus* with acutely branching septate hyphae that may invade blood vessels. Occasionally, macroconidia may be seen in tissue or draining cutaneous lesions. *Fusarium* species are common causes of keratitis and onychomycosis, but may also cause hematogenously disseminated mycoses in immunocompromised (usually neutropenic) patients. Blood cultures may be positive in approximately 70% of disseminated infections (in contrast to *Aspergillus*), and multiple cutaneous lesions are often seen. Treatment generally includes amphotericin B, but outcomes are poor unless the underlying immunosuppression is reversed. Newer approaches may include the newer triazoles, such as voriconazole or posaconazole (1,13).

Geophilic. Soil-associated dermatophytic fungi.

Geotrichum. A hyaline yeast-like organism, *Geotrichum* is characterized by true hyphae that segment into arthroconidia that are not separated by disjunctor cells. *Geotrichum* is found in soil, plants, air, water, sewage, and dairy products. It may also be found as normal flora in humans. It is an opportunistic pathogen that may cause mucosal and cutaneous infections and rarely fungemia and disseminated disease. Due to the rare nature of geotrichosis, the optimal treatment is unknown, but the organism appears susceptible to fluconazole, itraconazole, and the newer azoles, voriconazole and posaconazole.

Germ tube. A tubelike outgrowth from a conidium or spore; the beginning of a hypha with no constriction at the point of origin.

Gilchrist's disease. Another term for blastomycosis (1,11,12).

Gliocladium. A hyaline mold found in decaying vegetation and soil, *Gliocladium* is characterized by septate hyphae, branched conidiophores, and conidia that clump together in a cluster or ball. *Gliocladium* has not been documented to cause infection and is usually considered a contaminant when isolated in the laboratory.

Glucan. A structural carbohydrate of fungal cell walls.

Histoplasma capsulatum var. *capsulatum.* A thermally dimorphic pathogen endemic to the Ohio-

Mississippi River valleys, *H. capsulatum* is found in soil contaminated with bird or bat droppings. The organism grows as a small budding yeast in culture at 37°C and in tissue and as a mold with septate hyphae, large tuberculate macroconidia, and round microconidia in culture at 25°C and in nature. Infection is due to inhalation of conidia and is usually asymptomatic. Symptomatic disease may range from acute, self-limited pulmonary infection, to chronic, cavitary histoplasmosis, to disseminated disease. Treatment options include itraconazole or amphotericin B.

H. capsulatum var. *duboisii* occurs in periequatorial Africa. This organism is indistinguishable from var. *capsulatum* in vitro, but the yeast cells in tissue are considerably larger (8 to 15 μm versus 3 to 4 μm). Clinically, *H. capsulatum* var. *duboisii* causes focal bone and skin involvement and may cause fatal lymphoreticular disseminated disease.

Hormonema. *Hormonema* is a dematiaceous mold characterized by brown, thick-walled hyphae with cells wider than long. Hyaline blastoconidia emerge from dematiaceous hyphae. This organism is found in moist environments and causes wood-blueing of coniferous trees. It has been described as an agent of phaeohyphomycosis.

Hyaline. Nonpigmented structure.

Hypha. A filamentous structure of a fungus.

India ink. Stain used to highlight the capsule of *Cryptococcus neoformans* for detection in cerebrospinal fluid.

Internodal. The area of hypha between the sporangiophores of *Zygomycetes*.

Lasiodiplodia theobromae. A dematiaceous mold with broad septate, brown hyphae, *L. theobromae* belongs to the *Coelomycetes* and produces large, thick-walled striated conidia with a median septum within an asexual fruiting structure known as a pyncnidia. This organism is a tropical and subtropical plant pathogen and may cause keratitis, onychomycosis, and cutaneous and subcutaneous lesions.

Lecythophora. A hyaline mold found in soil and decaying vegetation, *Lecythophora* is characterized by septate hyphae with conidia produced in slimy heads. This organism has been implicated as an etiologic agent of keratitis and subcutaneous abscesses. It is susceptible to most antifungal agents, including amphotericin B and the azoles.

Macroconidium. The larger of two types of conidia in a fungus that produces both large and small conidia. May be either multicelled or single celled.

Malassezia. Yeast-like organisms that may be isolated from human skin (*M. furfur*) or from animals (*M. pachydermatis*), *Malassezia* spp. appear as budding yeast cells with small collarettes. Hyphae and pseudohyphae may be seen. *M. furfur* requires fatty acid supplementation for growth in vitro, whereas *M. pachydermatis* does not. *M. furfur* is the etiologic agent of pityriasis (tinea) versicolor, a superficial cutaneous mycosis, but may also cause catheter-related fungemia in patients receiving lipid supplementation. *M. pachydermatis* causes external otitis in dogs and has been implicated in catheter-related fungemias. Removal of the catheter is usually sufficient for treatment. Amphotericin B or fluconazole may be used in addition to catheter removal (1,9).

Malbranchea. A hyaline mold found in soil, decaying vegetable matter, and animal dung, *Malbranchia* is characterized by hyaline septate hyphae with arthroconidia separated by disjunctor cells. Gymnothecia containing ascospores may be formed in culture. The organism may be isolated from skin and nails but is not a recognized etiologic agent of mycotic disease.

Microascus. A dematiaceous mold found in soil and grain, *Microascus* is characterized by septate pigmented hyphae with conidia borne in chains. Perithecia containing asci and ascospores may be seen in culture. This organism is a rare cause of cutaneous infections. *M. cirrosus* has been reported to cause disseminated infection in a bone marrow transplant patient.

Microconidium. The smaller of two types of conidia in a fungus that produces both large and small conidia. It is usually single celled and rounded or ovoid in shape.

Microsporum. Dermatophytic molds characterized by numerous, thick-walled, septate macroconidia with accompanying microconidia, *Microsporum* species causing infections of scalp and skin include *M. audouinii, M. canis, M. cookei, M. gypseum, M. nanum,* and *M. gallinae. M. audouinii* is anthropophilic and is spread from human to human. *M. canis, M. nanum,* and *M. gallinae* are zoophilic, causing infection in animals with a secondary spread to humans. *M. cookei* and *M. gypseum* are geophilic, are found in soil, and may cause infection in both humans and animals. These organisms are generally responsive to treatment with azoles and/or terbinafine (3).

Mold. A fungus composed of filaments (hyphae) that generally form a colony that may be fuzzy, powdery, wooly, velvety, or smooth. Pigmentation may be present or absent and may vary from yellow, green, gray, black, brown, to red.

Mucor. Molds belonging to the class *Zygomycetes* in the order *Mucorales, Mucor* species are characterized by broad, sparsely septate, hyaline hyphae without rhizoids. They are found in soil and in decaying fruits and vegetables. *Mucor* spp. have been implicated as etiologic agents of rhinocerebral zygomycosis, sinusitis, and pulmonary and disseminated infections. As with other members of the *Zygomycetes, Mucor* spp. are opportunistic pathogens, and infections due to these agents are very difficult to manage without reconstitution of the host defense system. Antifungal therapy usually involves amphotericin B coupled with surgical resection of involved tissue whenever possible (5,14).

Muriform. Usually refers to a conidium having transverse and longitudinal septations.

Mycelium. A mat of intertwined hyphae that constitute the colony surface of a mold.

Mycetoma. Mycetoma refers to a mycotic infection that is chronic and characterized by indurated, swollen tissue with numerous draining sinuses. Mycetoma usually involves the lower extremities but may also involve the trunk. Over time, the mycetomatous process may involve bone and become disfiguring and destructive. Sinuses may drain purulent material containing granules of various shapes, pigmentation, and consistency. Eumycotic (true fungal) mycetoma may be caused by numerous fungi, both hyaline and dematiaceous. Response to anti-fungal therapy is usually poor because of the extent of disease at the time of diagnosis.

Mycosis. A disease caused by a fungus; including both yeasts and molds.

Mycotoxicosis. An intoxication, either local or systemic, due to a toxin produced by a fungus.

Nattrasia. A plant pathogen of tropical and sub-tropical locations, *Nattrasia* is a dematiaceous mold characterized by septate, pigmented hyphae of vary-ing widths, and formation of arthroconidia and phialoconidia. Arthroconidia are dark thick walled; they are not separated by disjunctor cells. This species is an etiologic agent of onychomycosis and dermato-mycosis involving soles and toe webs. Invasive disease has been described. Treatment includes amphotericin B (invasive disease) or azoles.

Onychomycosis. Local infection of a nail or nail bed (toe or finger) by a fungus (3).

Paecilomyces lilacinus. *P. lilacinus* is a hyaline mold characterized by septate hyphae and tapering phia-lides with chains of oblong conidia. Macroscopically, colonies have a faint lilac, violet, or mauve coloration. This organism is found in soil worldwide. Infections include keratitis and endophthalmitis, sinusitis, and catheter-related fungemia. This organism is relatively resistant to amphotericin B, but it has responded clinically to administration of ketoconazole and voriconazole.

Paracoccidioides brasiliensis. A dimorphic pathogenic fungus endemic to southern Mexico and Central and South America, this organism grows as a hyaline mold at 25°C in culture and in nature (soil, vegetation) and as a large spherical yeast with multiple buds arranged in the classical "mariner's wheel" at 37°C in tissue. Infection is manifested as a chronic granulomatous process involving lungs spreading to mucous membranes, skin, lymph nodes, and other organs. Treatment options include itraconazole, ketoconazole, amphotericin B, and trimethoprim/sulfamethoxazole (long-term suppression) (2).

Penicillium. A common, rapidly growing hyaline mold characterized by septate hyphae, branched conidiophores, and chains of conidia arranged in a "brush-like" configuration, *Penicillium* is a common contaminant that also may cause superficial and deep mycoses in its role as an opportunistic pathogen.

Penicillium marneffei. *P. marneffei* exhibits thermal dimorphism, growing as a mold at 25°C and as a yeast at 37°C and in tissue. The mold phase produces a characteristic diffusible red pigment. The yeast phase exhibits a central cross-wall as the cells multiply by fission rather than by budding. This organism is endemic in Southeast Asia and appears to have a zoonotic reservoir in the bamboo rat. Focal and disseminated infection mimicking histoplasmosis is seen in both immunocompetent and immunocompromised individuals. Positive blood cultures are not uncommon and are considered a marker of HIV infection in areas of endemicity. Infection is especially severe in individuals with AIDS. Treatment includes amphotericin B followed by itraconazole (1).

Perithecium. A large, rounded or pear-shaped structure having an ostiole (opening) and containing asci and ascospores.

Phaeoacremonium. A dematiaceous mold found in association with plants and characterized by dark septate hyphae and conidia arranged in round, slimy heads. *Phaeoacremonium* has been implicated in disseminated disease and as an agent of subcutaneous phaeohyphomycosis. Susceptibility to amphotericin B and the azoles is variable.

Phaeoannellomyces werneckii. A dematiaceous mold of tropical and subtropical regions, this organism is characterized by brown hyphae with prominent septa and one-and two-celled conidia. *P. werneckii* is the etiologic agent of tinea nigra and produces dark-pigmented lesions on the palms (usually only one palm) and the soles of the feet. The lesions are of cosmetic significance only, but they may resemble malignant melanoma and thus must be differentiated from this more serious condition.

Phaeohyphomycosis. Phaeohyphomycosis refers to mycotic infections caused by a variety of dematiaceous (dark-pigmented) fungi. The infection may be subcutaneous or systemic. In tissue, the fungal forms include both pigmented hyphae and yeast-like forms.

Phialide. A flask- or vase-shaped cell that produces conidia without tapering or increasing in length with each conidium produced.

Phialoconidium. Conidium produced at the end of a phialid.

Phialophora. A dematiaceous mold found in soil and decaying vegetation, *Phialophora* species are characterized by dark, septate, branching hyphae with flask-shaped phialides and round hyaline-to-brown conidia. *P. verrucosa* is the second most common agent of chromoblastomycosis, may also cause phaeohyphomycosis, and rarely, mycetoma. The other species, *P. richardsiae, P. repens,* and *P. parasitica* are etiologic agents of phaeohyphomycosis. Treatment includes surgery plus itraconazole or amphotericin B.

Phoma. *Phoma* is a dematiaceous mold characterized by brown, septate hyphae with occasional production of dark, thick-walled chlamydoconidia. Asexual fruiting bodies, pycnidia, containing slimy conidia, may be seen in culture. This organism is often considered a contaminant, but it has also been associated with keratitis and phaeohyphomycosis. It appears susceptible to itraconazole.

Pichia anomala (formerly *Hansenula anomala*). A yeast-like member of the *Ascomyetes*, *P. anomala* appears as a budding yeast with or without pseudo-hyphae. Asci containing hat- or helmet-shaped ascospores may be seen when cultured on ascospore medium. This organism is an opportunistic pathogen and has been reported to cause fungemia and endocarditis. It is considered susceptible to most antifungal agents, including azoles, amphotericin B, and flucytosine.

Pithium. A plant pathogen found in water and swampy environments, *Pithium* forms septate hyphae and may produce biflagellate motile zoospores. Disease in humans has been seen most commonly in Thailand and includes cutaneous and subcutaneous infection that may become angioinvasive. Keratitis and orbital cellulitis have also been reported. Optimal therapy has not been established; however, itraconazole combined with terbinafine may be efficacious.

Pithomyces. This dematiaceous mold has dark septate hyphae and conidia with either horizontal or muriform (horizontal and vertical) septa borne singly or in sporodochial arrays (clumps of conidiophores) in culture. Commonly considered a contaminant, *Pithomyces* has also been implicated as an opportunistic pathogen in immunocompromised individuals.

Pneumocystis carinii. Previously categorized as a protozoan parasite, *P. carinii* is now considered a fungus on the basis of recent molecular genetic evidence. *P. carinii* may appear in a trophic form, as a uninucleate sporocyst, or as a mature spore case or cyst containing up to eight oval to fusiform spores or intracystic bodies. Upon release of the intracystic bodies, the cyst wall may appear as empty oval or collapsed structures. *P. carinii* is an opportunistic pathogen that predominantly causes an interstitial pneumonitis in debilitated individuals (malnourished, infants, and the elderly) or immunocompromised individuals (with neutropenia, malignancies, or

AIDS). Extrapulmonary infections have also been described in individuals with AIDS. Diagnosis is made by staining pulmonary secretions with Gomori methenamine-silver, Giemsa, calcofluor, or fluorescent-labeled antibodies. Treatment options include trimethoprim/sulfamethoxazole or pentamidine. Prophylaxis with these agents may be useful in certain high-risk groups (e.g., leukemia, bone marrow transplant, AIDS) (15).

Prototheca wickerhamii. An achlorophyllous alga that appears yeast-like in culture and may be readily identified using commercial yeast identification systems. *P. wickerhami* demonstrates round sporangia of varying sizes containing sporangiospores. Neither budding nor hyphal formation occurs. This organism causes protothecosis, which may be cutaneous, subcutaneous, or systemic, depending on the host. Traumatic implantation is an important route of infection. Treatment includes surgical resection or debridement accompanied by administration of amphotericin B or itraconazole.

Pseudallescheria boydii. *P. boydii* is the sexual state of the fungus *Scedosporium apiospermum*. *P. boydii* is distinguished by the formation in culture of cleistothecia containing brown ascospores. The organism grows as a hyaline septate mold with a characteristic "mousy" gray color. *P. boydii* may cause mycetoma, pneumonia, meningitis and brain abscess, fungemia, and osteomyelitis. It is considered resistant to amphotericin B. Recently, dramatic responses to the newer triazoles, voriconazole and posaconazole, have been documented in patients with *Pseudallescheria* brain abscesses.

Pseudohypha. Chains of elongated cells formed by budding, which resembles a true hypha but is distinguished by constrictions at the septa, forming branches that begin with a septation and having terminal cells that are smaller than the other cells.

Pycnidium. A large, round or flask-shaped structure containing conidia and equipped with an opening or ostiole.

Ramichloridium mackenziei. A dematiaceous mold characterized by brown septate hyphae and pale-brown conidia, this organism is neurotropic and has been implicated in phaeohyphomycotic brain abscesses in patients from the Middle East. The organism is susceptible to amphotericin B, flucytosine, and the azoles.

Rhinocladiella. A dematiaceous mold found in decaying wood, *Rhinocladiella* is characterized by septate brown hyphae bearing unbranched conidiophores with ellipsoidal, closely packed conidia.

Disease in humans includes chromoblastomycosis, mycetoma, and central nervous system infection. Treatment includes surgical resection and antifungal therapy with amphotericin B or azoles.

Rhizoid. Branched, root-like structure located either directly beneath a sporangiophore (nodal) or between sporangiophores (internodal) of zygomycetes. Rhizoids extend into the culture medium.

Rhizomucor. A member of the class *Zygomycetes* in the order *Mucorales*, *Rhizomucor* is characterized by broad, hyaline, sparsely septate hyphae with branched sporangiophores and internodal rhizoids that are short and poorly developed. This organism is an etiologic agent of zygomycosis, including pulmonary, rhinocerebral, and disseminated disease. Zygomycosis due to this organism responds poorly to antifungal therapy (amphotericin B). Surgical resection of infected tissue is an important component of successful therapy (5,14).

Rhizopus. A rapidly growing member of the class *Zygomycetes* of the order *Mucorales*, *Rhizopus* is characterized by broad aseptate hyphae with unbranched sporangiophores and well developed rhizoids, which form immediately beneath the sporangiophores. *R. arrhizus* is the most common cause of zygomycosis. Rhinofacial and rhinocerebral diseases are often associated with uncontrolled diabetes and treatment with corticosteroids or iron chelation. Treatment includes administration of amphotericin B and surgical resection. The investigational triazole, posaconazole, exhibits promising activity against this organism and other agents of zygomycosis (5,14).

Rhodotorula rubra. A mucoid, pink- to red-pigmented budding yeast, *R. rubra* is urease positive and may appear weakly encapsulated. This organism may be isolated from skin and mucosal surfaces and has been implicated in peritonitis and fungemia, which is usually catheter related. *R. rubra* is susceptible to amphotericin B and flucytosine, but not to the azoles. Catheter removal is advised in cases of fungemia or peritonitis in patients undergoing peritoneal dialysis.

Saccharomyces cerevisiae. A urease-negative budding yeast, *S. cerevisiae* is a member of the class *Ascomycetes* and may form asci with ascospores when grown on special media. *S. cerevisiae* is found in numerous foods and may also colonize mucosal surfaces. Disease in humans is rare, but this yeast has been implicated in chronic vaginitis and fungemia. *S. cerevisiae* is usually susceptible to amphotericin B, flucytosine, and fluconazole.

Saksenaea vasiformis. A member of the class *Zygomycetes* in the order *Mucorales*, *S. vasiformis* has typical broad, hyaline, sparsely septate hyphae and characteristic flask- or vase-shaped sporangia. As with other members of the *Zygomycetes*, this organism is angioinvasive and may cause localized or disseminated zygomycosis. Surgical resection and administration of amphotericin B constitutes the treatment of choice (5,14).

Scedosporium apiospermum. See *Pseudallescheria boydii.*

Scedosporium prolificans. Formerly known as *S. inflatum*, *S. prolificans* is characterized by hyaline, septate hyphae, and basally inflated, flask-shaped conidiogenous cells with conidia borne in clumps. This organism has been implicated in a variety of infections following traumatic implantation; however, disseminated disease, which is almost uniformly fatal, has also been described. *S. prolificans* appears resistant to virtually all the systemically active antifungal agents. Limited success has been reported with the newly licensed triazole, voriconazole, coupled with surgical resection of infected tissue.

Schizophyllum commune. A member of the class *Basidiomycetes*, *S. commune* is a ubiquitous plant pathogen that may grow as a monokaryotic mold or, in the dikaryotic form, may go on to produce basidiocarps (mushrooms). Monokaryotic strains manifest both narrow and wider septate hyphae with lateral spicules. Dikaryotic strains demonstrate clamp connections at the point of septation. *S. commune* is a rare human pathogen, but it has been reported as the etiologic agent of oral ulcers, meningitis, brain abscess, sinusitis, and allergic bronchopulmonary mycosis. The organism appears to be susceptible to amphotericin B and itraconazole.

Scopulariopsis brevicaulis. A hyaline mold, *S. brevicaulis* is characterized by septate hyphae and thick-walled, spiny conidia borne in chains. This environmental mold may be associated with onycho-mycosis, cutaneous and soft-tissue infections, and rarely invasive pulmonary disease.

Scytalidium. This genus contains both hyaline (moniliaceous) and dematiaceous molds. The hyaline form is *S. hyalinium* and its dematiaceous counterpart is *S. dimidiatum*. These molds produce septate hyphae and single-celled arthroconidia that are not separated by disjunctor cells. Both species may cause clinical disease, including onychomycosis, cutaneous infections, and rarely more invasive disease. Susceptibility to amphotericin B and the azoles has been documented.

Septum. Cross-wall within hyphae or between fungal cells.

Sporangiophore. A specialized hyphal structure bearing a sporangium.

Sporangiospore. An asexual spore produced within a sporangium.

Sporangium. A closed, sac-like structure in which asexual spores (sporangiospores) are produced by cleavage.

Sporobolomyces salmonicolor. A yeast-like fungus that produces salmon pink- or coral-colored colonies on culture, this organism is urease positive and forms both true hyphae and pseudohyphae from sickle-shaped ballistospores. Ballistospores are formed on denticles and are forcibly discharged forming satellite colonies on the culture plate. This organism rarely causes infection but has been isolated from blood, urine, and sputum.

Sporothrix schenckii. A thermally dimorphic fungus growing as a mold in culture at 25°C and in nature and as a yeast at 37°C in tissue. The mold form demonstrates hyaline septate hyphae with hyaline conidia arranged in a rosette, and larger, thick-walled brown conidia that are attached directly to the hyphae. The yeast form is rarely seen in tissue but may be round, oval, or "cigar-shaped" with single or multiple buds. *S. schenckii* may be found in soil and decaying vegetation and causes characteristic lymphocutaneous lesions following traumatic implantation. Pulmonary, laryngeal, and hematogenous forms of sporotrichosis may also occur but are much less common than the lymphocutaneous form. Itraconazole has displaced potassium iodide for treatment of lymphocutaneous infection. Amphotericin B is recommended for treatment of disseminated and meningeal infection.

Sporotrichum. An environmental mold characterized by broad septate hyphae with occasional clamp connections, single-celled, thick-walled conidia and large, thick-walled chlamydoconidia. This organism is usually considered to be a contaminant when isolated in culture, but it may cause pulmonary disease.

Stachybotrys. An environmental mold that produces hyaline to pigmented septate hyphae and dark oval conidia that form in clusters, *Stachybotrys* produces a toxin that may be lethal to animals on ingestion. It has also been implicated in numerous cases of "sick building" syndrome in recent years, possibly secondary to inhalation of toxin and/or spores by human inhabitants of buildings or houses contaminated by the mold.

Syncephalastrum racemosum. A species of the class *Zygomycetes* in the order *Mucorales*, *S. racemosum* demonstrates typical broad, hyaline, sparsely septate hyphae with rhizoids. The sporangial heads are composed of tubular sacs containing up to 10 sporangiospores. This organism has rarely been implicated in disease in humans. As with other members of *Zygomycetes*, *S. racemosum* appears susceptible to amphotericin B but resistant to the azoles.

Teleomorph. The sexual form of a conidiogenous fungus.

Thermal dimorphism. Ability of a fungus to switch between a yeast (37°C) and a mold (25°C) form with changes in temperature.

Trichoderma. An environmental mold that only recently has been implicated in infections in humans. *Trichoderma* manifests hyaline septate hyphae and round, green-pigmented conidia borne in clusters. Macroscopically, the colony is characterized by blue-green or yellow-green coloration. This is an opportunistic pathogen and has caused fatal disseminated infection in immunocompromised individuals. Susceptibility to amphotericin B appears variable, and the organism does not appear to be susceptible to the azoles.

Trichophyton. *Trichophyton* are dermatophytic molds characterized by numerous microconidia and rare multicelled macroconidia. Several species are known human pathogens, including *T. rubrum, T. mentagrophytes, T. tonsurans, T. verrucosum, T. schoenleini,* and *T. violaceum. T. rubrum* is the most common dermatophyte to infect humans. Sites of infection include skin, nails, and hair. Treatment options include the azoles (itraconazole, ketoconazole, fluconazole), terbinafine, and griseofulvin.

Trichosporon. Yeast-like fungi characterized by budding yeast (blastocondidia), true hyphae, and pseudohyphae. Arthroconidia without disjunctor cells are also prominent. *T. beigelii (cutanium)* is the most common cause of systemic or disseminated disease among the various species of this genus. Infection of the hair shafts (white piedra) is seen in tropical countries. Deep infections include endocarditis, meningitis, and peritonitis, as well as hematogenous dissemination in immunocompromised individuals. *Trichosporon* species may be resistant to amphotericin B, but are usually susceptible to the azoles and flucytosine.

Ulocladium. A dematiaceous mold found in soil and decaying plants. *Ulocladium* is characterized by brown septate hyphae and brown-to-black, rough conidia with both transverse and longitudinal septations. This organism is a rare cause of subcutaneous phaeohyphomycosis. Treatment is similar to that of other phaeohyphomycotic infections and includes surgery, amphotericin B, and itraconazole.

Ustilago. A yeast-like member of the class *Basidiomycetes*, *Ustilago* is characterized by elongate, spindle-shaped, yeast-like cells that produce hyphae with clamp connections. This organism is a plant pathogen and may be rarely isolated from clinical specimens such as sputum. Its role in any human disease process is unclear.

Verticillium. A hyaline mold with septate hyphae and conidiophores that may be branched and arranged in whorls (verticillate). Conidia may be single or in clusters. This organism is found in soil and decaying vegetation and may cause keratitis. Its role in other disease processes is uncertain.

Vesicle. Enlarged structure at the end of a conidiophore or sporangiophore.

Zoophilic. A dermatophytic fungus that infects both animals and humans.

Zygomycosis. A disease process involving one of a number of the class *Zygomycetes* in the order *Mucorales*, including *Absidia*, *Cunninghamella*, *Mucor*, *Rhizopus*, *Rhizomucor*, and *Saksenaea*, among others. Zygomycosis is marked by angioinvasion by the fungal hyphae with subsequent infarction and tissue destruction. It occurs predominantly in patients who are compromised by diabetes, leukemia, or bone marrow and solid organ transplantation. It may involve lungs, sinuses, brain, or skin, or it may be widely disseminated. Treatment involves surgical resection of the infected tissue and administration of amphotericin B, as well as efforts to reverse or control the underlying predisposing disease process. Posaconazole, an investigational triazole, may have some activity against the etiologic agents of zygomycosis (5,14).

REFERENCES

1. **Anaissie, E. J., M. R. McGinnis, and M. A. Pfaller.** 2003. *Clinical Mycology.* Churchill Livingstone, Philadelphia, Pa.

2. **Brummer, E., E. Castaneda, and A. Restrepo.** 1993. Paracoccidioidomycosis: an update. *Clin. Microbiol. Rev.* 6:89–117.

3. **Elewski, B. E.** 1998. Onychomycosis: pathogenesis, diagnosis, and management. *Clin. Microbiol. Rev.* 11:415–429.

4. **Fidel, P. L., Jr., J. A. Vazquez, and J. D. Sobel.** 1999. *Candida glabrata:* review of epidemiology, pathogenesis, and clinical disease with comparison to *C. albicans. Clin. Microbiol. Rev.* 12:80–96.

5. **Gonzalez, C. E., M. G. Rinaldi, and A. M. Sugar.** 2002. Zygomycosis. *Infect. Dis. Clin N. Am.* 16:895–914.

6. **Hazen, K. C.** 1995. New and emerging yeast pathogens. *Clin. Microbiol. Rev.* **8:**462–478.

7. **Larone, D. H.** 2002. *Medically Important Fungi: a Guide to Identification*, 4th ed. ASM Press, Washington, D.C.

8. **Latge, J.-P.** 1999. *Aspergillus fumigatus* and aspergillosis. *Clin. Microbiol. Rev.* **12:**310–350.

9. **Marcon, M. J., and D. A. Powell.** 1992. Human infections due to *Malassezia* spp. *Clin. Microbiol. Rev.* **5:**101–119.

10. **Marr, K. A., T. Patterson, and D. Denning.** 2002. Aspergillosis: pathogenesis, clinical manifestations, and therapy. *Infect. Dis. Clin. N. Am.* **16:**875–894.

11. **Mujeeb, I., D. A. Sutton, A. W. Fothergill, M. G. Rinaldi, and M. A. Pfaller.** 2002. Fungi and fungal infections, p. 1125–1156. *In* K. D. McClatchey (ed.), *Clinical Laboratory Medicine*, 2nd ed. Lippincott Williams & Wilkins, Philadelphia, Pa.

12. **Murray, P. R., E. J. Baron, J. H. Jorgensen, M. A. Pfaller, and R. H. Yolken.** 2003. *Manual of Clinical Microbiology*, 8th ed. ASM Press, Washington, D.C.

13. **Nelson, P. E., M. C. Dignani, and E. J. Anaissie.** 1994. Taxonomy, biology, and clinical aspects of *Fusarium* species. *Clin. Microbiol. Rev.* **7:**479–504.

14. **Ribes, J. A., C. L. Vanover-Sama, and D. J. Boker.** 2002. Zygomycetes in human disease. *Clin. Microbiol. Rev.* **13:**236–301.

15. **Stringer, J. R.** 1996. *Pneumocystis carinii:* what is it, exactly? *Clin. Microbiol. Rev.* **9:**489–498.

Parasites

Acanthamoeba. Opportunistic free-living amebae found in soil and water. The organism is characterized by spike-like pseudopods (acanthopodia), formation of round wrinkled uninucleate cysts, and the lack of a flagellate state. Infections include chronic granulomatous amebic encephalitis (GAE), meningoencephalitis (rare), keratitis, and endophthalmitis. Hematogenous dissemination may occur with resultant granulomatous infection of skin, bone, and other tissues. Nine species of *Acanthamoeba* have been identified from infections in humans. *A. castellani* is the most common species, causing GAE and ocular infections, followed by *A. culbertsoni* (GAE) and *A. polyphaga* (ocular infections). Diagnosis is usually made by microscopic examination of tissue biopsy material or corneal scrapings; however, culture may be also be useful.

Amastigote. The rounded intracellular form of hemoflagellates of the genus *Trypanosoma* and *Leishmania*. The amastigote stage of these organisms is always intracellular and lacks the undulating membrane and external flagellum seen in other stages. The only structures that can be distinguished in this stage are the nucleus and the kinetoplast.

Amebae. Simple unicellular protozoan parasites that exist in two stages, a motile feeding stage (trophozoite) and a dormant, resistant, infective stage (cyst). The trophozoite form uses cytoplasmic extrusions or pseudopods as a means of motility. The organism assumes the cyst form in response to unfavorable environmental conditions. Most amebae found in humans are nonpathogenic commensals (*Entamoeba coli*, *Entamoeba hartmanii*, *Entamoeba dispar*, *Entamoeba gingivalis*, *Endolimax nana*, and *Iodamoeba bütschlii*). *Entamoeba histolytica* is an important human pathogen as are the opportunistic free-living amebae (*Naegleria*, *Acanthamoeba*, *Balamuthia*) that are found in water and soil.

Amebiasis. An infectious process caused by *E. histolytica* that may be either intestinal or extraintestinal in nature. Intestinal amebiasis produces clinical signs and symptoms of abdominal pain, cramping, and diarrhea related to localized tissue destruction produced by the organism in the large intestine. Extraintestinal amebiasis most commonly involves the liver with abscess formation and systemic signs of infection (fever, chills, leukocytosis). An asymptomatic intestinal carrier state may also be seen with *E. histolytica* or the noninvasive *E. dispar*.

Ancylostoma. A genus of nematode (roundworm) referred to as a hookworm.

    A. braziliense. A species of hookworm that is a natural parasite of dogs and cats. Infection in humans with this species is accidental and results in serpentine cutaneous lesions that may be quite erythematous and pruritic (cutaneous larva migrans). The filariform larvae of this species can penetrate human skin but are unable to develop further. Although irritating, the infection is self-limited and requires symptomatic treatment only. Diagnosis is usually made based on the characteristic skin lesions and a history of contact with dog and/or cat feces.

    A. duodenale. A hookworm that parasitizes the small intestine in humans and may produce gastrointestinal symptoms of nausea, vomiting, and diarrhea, as well as anemia due to chronic blood loss. Eggs are shed in feces and develop in the soil into infectious filariform larvae, which can then penetrate exposed skin and initiate a new cycle of infection. Infections occur primarily in warm subtropical and tropical regions and in the southern regions of the United States. Diagnosis of infection due to *A. duodenale* in humans is made by microscopic examination of stool.

Angiostrongylus cantonensis. A tissue-dwelling nematode, *A. cantonensis* is also known as the rat-lung worm. It has a wide distribution in the tropics and subtropics, where its life cycle involves molluscs (larval stage in slugs and snails) and rats (adult stage). In human hosts, *A. cantonensis* does not complete its development cycle. When the infective larvae are ingested, they migrate from the intestinal tract to the meninges and remain there rather than continuing on to the lungs as they do in rats. The subsequent death of the larvae in the meninges sets up a profound inflammatory reaction resulting in human eosinophilic meningitis. In areas of endemicity a presumptive diagnosis may be made on the basis of meningitis with blood and spinal fluid eosinophila. Most patients recover uneventfully with symptomatic and supportive care.

Ascaris lumbricoides. This large (20 to 35 cm long) intestinal roundworm is found in temperate and tropical areas worldwide. Superficially, it resembles an earthworm; however, it has a tough external cuticle that is creamy white in color. Infection in

humans results when eggs are ingested with
contaminated soil or food. The eggs hatch in the
duodenum, and the larvae migrate to the lungs and
eventually find their way back to the small bowel
where they mature and begin producing large
numbers of eggs. Most infections are asymptomatic;
however, large numbers of worms may result in vague
abdominal complaints and occasionally in bowel
obstruction. Adult worms generally remain in the
small bowel, but they may migrate into the pancreas,
bile ducts, and liver with severe consequences. Tissue
migration of larvae and adult worms is generally
accompanied by a moderate eosinophilia. Microscopic examination of stool will reveal the characteristic eggs; however, the diagnosis is often made
visually when the worms are passed into the stool.

Babesia. Members of the genus *Babesia* are intra-
erythrocytic protozoan parasites. Humans are
infected when bitten by an infected tick. The parasites
multiply within red blood cells, eventually lysing the
cells, with subsequent infection of additional cells to
maintain the infection. *B. microti* is the most common
agent of babesiosis in the United States, whereas
B. divergens has been reported more frequently in
Europe. Most infections are mild or asymptomatic,
but severe, often fatal, infections may be seen in
asplenic individuals. Microscopic examination of

Giemsa-stained blood smears is the diagnostic method of choice (4).

Balamuthia mandrillaris. Another genus of free-living amebae found in soil and water. As with *Acanthamoeba* species, *Balamuthia* causes chronic granulomatous amebic encephalitis and brain abscesses, primarily in immunocompromised individuals. Both amebic trophozoites and cysts may be found in infected tissue, and the trophozoites may also be detected in cerebrospinal fluid.

Balantidium coli. An intestinal protozoan, *B. coli* is the only member of the ciliate group that is pathogenic for humans. *B. coli* is a large (50 to 200 μm long and 40 to 70 μm wide) ciliated protozoan that may exist as a motile trophozoite or in a cyst form. The organism causes gastrointestinal disease similar to amebiasis with ulceration of the intestinal mucosa and associated abdominal pain, nausea, and bloody diarrhea. *B. coli* is a parasite of pigs and is found worldwide. Infections are transmitted by the fecal-oral route and are associated with contamination of water and food supplies with pig feces. Diagnosis is made by microscopic detection of trophozoites and cysts in fecal material.

Bancroft's filariasis. An infection of the lymphatic system due to the nematode *Wuchereria bancrofti*. It occurs in tropical and subtropical areas throughout the world and is marked by fever, eosinophilia, lymphangitis, and lymphadenopathy. Ultimately, tremendous lymphedema and tissue damage lead to the condition known as elephantiasis.

Beef tapeworm. See *Taenia saginata*.

Biharziasis. Disease caused by various species of schistosomes: *Schistosoma mansoni, S. japonicum,* and *S. haematobium*. Also known as schistosomiasis or snail fever. See *Schistosoma* for additional details.

Blackwater fever. Kidney damage associated with *Plasmodium falciparum* malaria, results in a constellation of signs and symptoms known as blackwater fever. Intravascular hemolysis due to massive destruction of both infected and uninfected red blood cells produces hemoglobinuria and can result in acute renal failure, tubular necrosis, nephrotic syndrome, and death. Liver involvement may also be seen and is characterized by abdominal pain, vomiting of bile, severe diarrhea, and dehydration (9).

Bladder worm. Another term for the cysticercus larval stage of tapeworms of the genus *Taenia*. This stage is found in tissue of an infected host and consists of a fluid-filled bladder with a single scolex or attachment organ equipped with hooklets.

Blastocystis hominis. An intestinal ameba of unde-termined pathogenicity. *B. hominis* may be found equally in individuals with and without gastrointes-tinal symptoms. It has been suggested that large numbers of *B. hominis* present in stools of immuno-compromised individuals may be significant; how-ever, the definitive role of this organism in gastrointestinal disease remains to be demonstrated (10).

Blood flukes. See *Schistosoma*.

Brugia malayi. The agent of Malayan filariasis, *B. malayi* is a nematode that parasitizes the lymphatic system of infected individuals in the Asia Pacific region of the world. A mosquito vector introduces infective third-stage larvae via a bite wound. The larvae migrate to the lymphatics where they grow to adulthood. The adults produce sheathed microfilar-iae, which gain access to the circulation where they then may infect feeding mosquitoes. The sheathed microfilaria is the diagnostic form of the organism and may be detected by microscopic examination of Giemsa-stained blood films. Greater numbers of microfilariae are present in the circulation at night (10 p.m. to 4 a.m.; nocturnal periodicity). Clinical disease is caused by obstruction of the lymphatics by the adult worms coupled with recurrent inflamma-tion, resulting in the clinical picture of elephantiasis.

Calabar swellings. Transient subcutaneous swellings, usually on the extremities, produced as adult *Loa loa* worms migrate through subcutaneous tissue. The swellings are large, nodular areas that are painful and pruritic. Because eosinophilia (50 to 70%) is observed, calabar swellings are considered to be secondary to an allergic reaction to the worms or their metabolic products.

Cercariae. Motile ciliated larval forms of schistosome flukes that are found free-swimming in freshwater. Cercariae are the infective form of schistosomes that penetrate intact skin, enter the circulation, and mature in the intrahepatic portal circulation.

Cercarial dermatitis. An intensely pruritic skin rash associated with immediate- and delayed-type hypersensitivity to parasite antigens that occurs following skin penetration by schistosome cercariae. Also known as "swimmer's itch," cercarial dermatitis may occur following exposure to the cercariae of avian schistosomes as well as schistosomes of humans.

Cestodes. Also known as tapeworms, cestodes have bodies composed of segments, or proglottids. All cestodes are hermaphroditic, and all lack digestive systems; nutrition is absorbed through the body walls. Each proglottid contains a complete set of reproductive organs. The life cycles of some cestodes are simple and direct, whereas those of others are complex and require one or more intermediate hosts.

Chagas' disease. Also known as American trypanosomiasis, Chagas' disease is caused by *Trypanosoma cruzi*. Infection is initiated by the bite of a reduviid bug. Organisms in the feces of the bug enter the wound and migrate to other tissues (e.g., cardiac muscle, liver, brain), where they assume the amastigote stage, multiply intracellularly, and eventually destroy the host cells. Acute infection is marked by fever, chills, malaise, myalgia, and fatigue. Acute central nervous system involvement is often seen in children. Chronic Chagas' disease is characterized by hepatomegaly, myocarditis, and enlargement of the esophagus and colon as a result of the destruction of nerve cells and other tissues that control the growth of these organs. Death from chronic Chagas' disease results from tissue destruction in the many areas invaded by the organisms, and sudden death results from complete heart block and brain damage.

Chagoma. An area of erythema and induration surrounding the bite of a reduviid bug. This is considered one of the earliest signs of Chagas' disease and is often followed by a rash and edema of the surrounding area.

Ciliates. Includes a variety of free-living and symbiotic species of motile protozoa. Ciliate locomotion involves the coordinated movement of rows of hair-like structures, or cilia. Cilia are similar in structure to flagella but are usually shorter and more numerous. Some ciliates are multinucleate. *Balantidium coli*, the only ciliate parasite of humans, contains two nuclei: a large macronucleus and a small micronucleus.

Clonorchis sinensis. See *Opisthorchis sinensis*.

Coccidia. Also referred to as *Sporozoa*. Unicellular organisms of the phylum Apicomplexa, which include both intestinal parasites (e.g., *Cryptosporidium* and *Cyclospora* species) and blood and tissue parasites (e.g., *Plasmodium, Babesia*, and *Toxoplasma* species). Coccidia have a system of organelles at their apical end that produces substances that facilitate penetration of host cells by the organism. Other typical characteristics include the existence of both asexual (schizogony) and sexual (gametogony) reproduction. Most members of the group also share alternative hosts; for example, in malaria, mosquitoes harbor the sexual cycle and humans harbor the asexual cycle.

Creeping eruption. Also known as *ground itch* or *cutaneous larva migrans*. Creeping eruption is caused by the filariform larva of *Ancylostoma braziliense*, the dog and cat hookworm. When humans come into contact with soil contaminated with feces of infected animals, the filariform larvae present in the soil penetrate the skin but are unable to develop further. The larvae remain "trapped" in the wrong host for weeks to months and wander through the subcutaneous tissues, creating serpentine tunnels. The migrating larvae provoke a severe erythematous and vesicular reaction in the skin. Pruritis and scratching of the involved skin may lead to secondary bacterial infection.

Cryptosporidium parvum. A coccidian parasite that is distributed worldwide, *C. parvum* causes gastrointestinal disease that is usually self-limited. Waterborne transmission of cryptosporidiosis has been well documented as an important route of infection. Disease in previously healthy individuals is usually a mild, self-limited enterocolitis characterized by watery diarrhea without blood. In contrast, disease in individuals with AIDS may be severe, with 50 or more stools per day causing tremendous fluid loss, and can last from months to years. Diagnosis is made by microscopic examination of fecal specimens using a modified acid-fast stain or an indirect immunofluorescence assay (5).

Cutaneous larva migrans. See Creeping eruption.

Cyclospora cayetanensis. Like *C. parvum*, *C. cayetanensis* is a water-borne coccidian parasite that causes diarrheal disease in individuals worldwide. Clinical symptoms include nausea, anorexia, abdominal cramping, and watery diarrhea. The diarrhea is usually self-limited in immunocompetent hosts and severe and prolonged in immunocompromised individuals. The diagnosis is based on microscopic detection of oocysts in stool. Currently, there are no immunodiagnostic methods to aid in the diagnosis and monitoring of this infection.

Cysticercosis. A human infection with the larval form of *Taenia solium*, the cysticerci, which normally infects pigs. Ingestion of water or vegetation contaminated with *T. solium* eggs initiates the infection. Once ingested, the eggs hatch, releasing an oncosphere, which penetrates the intestinal wall and migrates through the circulation to various tissues where it develops into a cysticercus, or bladder worm. The cysticerci may develop in muscle, connective tissue, brain, lungs, and eyes, and remain viable for as long as 5 years. The enlarging cysticerci may cause signs and symptoms of a space-occupying lesion producing hydrocephalus, seizures, and visual defects. Cerebral cysticercosis is especially common in individuals from Mexico. Diagnosis is usually made by radiographic visualization of the mass and/or detection of cysticerci in tissue removed surgically.

Cysticercus. See Bladder worm and Cysticercosis, above.

Delhi boil. The skin lesion seen in cutaneous leishmaniasis caused by *Leishmania tropica* is commonly referred to as *Delhi boil* or *Oriental sore*. The site of a bite from a sandfly infected with *L. tropica* appears as a red papule, which gradually enlarges and ulcerates. Eventually, the ulcer becomes hard and crusted and exudes a thin serous material. The amastigote form of the organism may be seen in properly stained smears from touch preparations of ulcer biopsy specimens. The lesion may heal without treatment over a period of months, but usually leaves a disfiguring scar.

Dientamoeba fragilis. A protozoan parasite that is classified as a flagellate, *D. fragilis* has no cyst state. *D. fragilis* is an intestinal parasite with worldwide distribution. Most infections are asymptomatic, but some patients may develop abdominal discomfort, flatulence, diarrhea, anorexia, and weight loss. There is no evidence that *D. fragilis* invades tissue. The diagnosis is made by microscopic examination of stool.

Diphyllobothrium latum. Also known as the "fish tapeworm," *D. latum* is a large (20 to 30 feet long) tapeworm that occurs worldwide. It has a complex life cycle that involves two intermediate hosts: fresh-water crustaceans and freshwater fish. Ingestion of the second stage larvae, or sparaganum, in uncooked or poorly cooked fish initiates infection in humans. The tapeworm attaches to the wall of the small intestine by its scolex, which does not have hooklets, and grows by developing proglottids. Eggs are produced in the proglottids and are shed in the stool. Eggs may be produced at a rate of more than 1 million per day over a period of months to years. On reaching freshwater, the eggs hatch and the free-swimming larva, or coracidium, is ingested by crustaceans known as copepods. The larval stage develops in the copepod, which is then eaten by a fish, and the sparaganum larvae develop in the musculature of the fish. Most *D. latum* infections are asymptomatic; however, a small percentage (0.1 to 2%) of people infected with this organism develop signs and symptoms of vitamin B_{12} deficiency. Diagnosis is made by recovering proglottids and/or eggs in the stool of infected individuals.

Dipylidium caninum. Commonly referred to as the "pumpkinseed tapeworm." A small (15 cm) tape-worm, it is primarily a parasite of dogs and cats. Humans may become infected when licked on the mouth by infected pets. The life cycle involves the development of larval worms in dog and cat fleas, which are then ingested, leading to intestinal infection. The organism is found worldwide and transmission is directly correlated with dogs and cats infected with fleas. Light infections are usually asymptomatic, whereas heavy infections produce abdominal discomfort, anal pruritis, and diarrhea. Stool examination reveals packets of eggs, and proglottids may be seen macroscopically.

Dirofilaria immitis. Also known as dog heartworm, *D. immitis* is a filarial nematode that is transmitted by mosquitoes to dogs and may occasionally be found in humans. In dogs, the adult worms develop in the chambers of the heart and may form a lethal worm bolus. In humans, this nematode does not complete its life cycle but may lodge in the lung, forming an asymptomatic coin lesion that may be mistaken for malignancy upon radiographic examination.

Dracunculus medinensis. A tissue-invading nematode of clinical importance in many parts of Asia and equatorial Africa. The life cycle of *D. medinensis* includes freshwater and a copepod of the genus *Cyclops.* Drinking contaminated water results in ingestion of *Cyclops* bearing larval *D. medinensis*, liberation of larvae in the stomach, penetration of the wall of the digestive tract, and subsequent migration of larvae to the retroperitoneal space where they mature. Male and female worms mate in the retroperitoneum and the fertilized female then migrates to the subcutaneous tissues, usually in the lower extremities. When the fertilized female becomes gravid, a vesicle forms on the surface of the skin which then ulcerates. The worm protrudes a loop of uterus through the ulcer and upon contact with water the larval forms are released. Symptoms are generally confined to the site of the ulcer and consist of pain and erythema. Secondary bacterial infection may lead to further tissue destruction and inflammation.

Dumdum fever. Also known as kala-azar, dumdum fever refers to the clinical picture of visceral leishmaniasis due to *Leishmania donovani*. This infection occurs in many parts of Asia, Africa, and Southeast Asia. Symptoms include chills and fever that may resemble that of malaria. As organisms proliferate and invade cells of the liver and spleen, marked hepatosplenomegaly, weight loss, and emaciation occur. If untreated, visceral leishmaniasis develops into an acute fulminating lethal disease or may persist as a chronic debilitating disease, leading to death within 1 to 2 years.

Echinococcus. This genus includes two species of tapeworm, *E. granulosus* and *E. multilocularis*, that cause accidental infections in humans. The adult form of *E. granulosus* occurs in canines (dogs, wolves, coyotes), and the larval cyst stage occurs in herbivores. The adult tapeworm consists of a *Taenia*-like scolex with four sucking disks and hooklets, as well as three proglottids, one of which contains eggs. The eggs are passed in the feces and ingestion of eggs by a human results in release of the larvae, which penetrate the digestive tract and are carried by the circulation to various tissues (brain, bone, liver, lungs). In the tissue, the larvae form unilocular cysts, which are slow-growing tumor-like structures enclosed by a laminated germinative membrane. The membrane produces structures on its wall called brood capsules, where tapeworm heads (protoscolices) develop. Daughter cysts may develop within the mother cyst and produce brood capsules. The cysts expand and accumulate fluid as they grow. Symptoms occur gradually over a period of years and are usually related to the space-occupying nature of the expanding cyst within the organ. Rupture of cysts produces fever, rash, and occasionally anaphylactic shock and death. The release of thousands of brood capsules and proto-scolices leads to dissemination of the infection.

Infection with *E. multilocularis* is very similar to that of *E. granulosus*. The cyst of *E. multilocularis* develops as an alveolar or honeycombed structure that is not covered by a limiting membrane. The cyst grows by exogenous budding, eventually resembling a carcinoma. As with *E. granulosus*, symptomatology is due to the space-occupying cyst mass within an organ.

Infection with *E. granulosus* in humans occurs in sheep-raising countries such as Europe, South America, Africa, Asia, Australia, and New Zealand. *E. multilocularis* is found in northern areas such as Canada, Russia, northern Japan, Central Europe, Alaska, Montana, North and South Dakota, Minnesota, and Iowa.

Elephantiasis. A condition that usually involves the lower extremities with massive swelling and lymphedema secondary to the presence of filarial worms in the lymphatics. Blockage of lymph flow by the physical presence of the worms coupled with chronic inflammation results in pooling and extravasation of lymphatic fluid plus tremendous scarring and fibrosis of the surrounding tissues. The worms most commonly involved are *Brugia malayia* and *Wuchereria bancrofti*. See Bancroft's filariasis.

Encephalitozoon. Formerly known as *Septata*, this genus of microsporidia includes three species, *E. hellem, E. cuniculi,* and *E. intestinalis.* All are obligate intracellular pathogens that may cause chronic diarrhea, ocular and neurologic infections, and hepatitis. See Microsporidia (2).

Entamoeba. A genus of protozoan parasites that includes *E. histolytica, E. coli, E. dispar,* and *E. gingivalis. Entamoeba* species may exist in an

ameboid trophic state or an infectious dormant cyst
state. See Amebae and Amebiasis.

Enterobius vermicularis. Also known as pinworm,
E. vermicularis is a small white worm that parasitizes
the large intestine and perianal area of infected
individuals. *E. vermicularis* occurs worldwide and is
spread by fecal-oral contact. Ingestion of eggs results
in infection of the distal large bowel. The gravid
female worm migrates to the perianal folds and
deposits large numbers of eggs, which are infectious
within hours. The eggs can survive for long periods
outside the host, resulting in recurrent cycles of
infection. Signs and symptoms may be absent but
most commonly present as pruritis of the perianal
region. Worms may migrate to the vagina and
produce genitourinary problems. Detection of characteristic eggs by microscopic examination of an anal
swab or "scotch-tape" specimen provides diagnostic
confirmation.

Enterocytozoon bieneusi. A species of microsporidia
that is best known as a cause of chronic diarrhea in
patients with AIDS, *E. bieneusi* is an obligate intracellular pathogen. See Microsporidia (2).

Espundia. Also known as chiclero ulcer, espundia is a
common name for mucocutaneous leishmaniasis due
to *Leishmania braziliensis*. This infection is seen from

the Yucatan peninsula into Central and South America, especially in the rain forests where workers are exposed to sandfly bites. As the name implies, the clinical disease is marked by involvement and destruction of mucous membranes and related tissue structures of the nares and oropharynx. Resulting edema and secondary bacterial infection produce severe and disfiguring facial mutilation.

Fasciola hepatica. Commonly called the sheep liver fluke, *F. hepatica* is a trematode (fluke) that parasitizes herbivores (primarily sheep and cattle) and humans. Infection in humans results from ingestion of plants (watercress) that harbor the encysted larval form or metacercaria. The infective larval fluke migrates through the wall of the duodenum, across the peritoneal cavity, and into the liver, where it matures within the bile ducts. Adults are large, flat leaf-shaped worms equipped with attachment suckers and both male and female reproductive organs (hermaphroditic). Mature adults produce operculated eggs that pass with the bile into the bowel and are excreted in the stool of the infected host. Mechanical and chemical irritation of the bile ducts caused by the adult flukes may produce hepatitis, hyperplasia of the epithelium, and biliary obstruction. Invasion of the liver parenchyma produces necrosis or "liver rot." The laboratory diagnosis is made by detecting the operculated eggs on microscopic examination of stool.

Fasciolopsis buski. The largest and most common of the intestinal flukes, *F. buski* has a life cycle similar to *Fasciola hepatica* in that the larvae undergo development in freshwater snails, encyst on aquatic vegetation, and infect humans/animals upon ingestion of the vegetation. The metacercariae develop into mature flukes within the small intestine and undergo self-fertilization. The operculated eggs are indistinguishable from those of *F. hepatica* and are passed in the stool. The symptoms of *F. buski* infection relate directly to the worm burden in the small intestine. Severe infections produce abdominal discomfort and diarrhea. The attachment of the fluke to the intestinal mucosa can produce inflammation, ulceration, and bleeding.

Filariasis. Infection due to one of a number of nematodes that produce filariform larvae, including *Wuchereria bancrofti, Brugia malayi, Loa loa, Onchocerca volvulus, Mansonella perstans, Mansonella streptocerca,* and *Mansonella ozzardi*. Most commonly seen in tropical and subtropical regions of the world, infections due to these organisms are often marked by fever, eosinophilia, lymphangitis, and lymphadenopathy. Infections due to *W. bancrofti* and *B. malayi* often produce elephantiasis, whereas

O. volvulus may cause blindness secondary to migration of microfilariae through the eyes.

Fish tapeworm. See *Diphyllobothrium latum*.

Flagellates. Unicellular protozoan parasites that move by the lashing of their whip-like flagella. The number and position of flagella may vary with different species. Specialized structures associated with the flagella may produce a characteristic appearance that may be useful in species identification. Examples of flagellates include *Leishmania* spp., *Trypanosoma* spp., *Trichomonas* spp., and *Giardia* spp.

Flatworms. Worms belonging to the phylum Platyhelminthes. Flatworms have flattened bodies that are leaf-like or resemble ribbon segments. Platyhelminthes can be further divided into trematodes (flukes) and cestodes (tapeworms). Trematodes have leaf-shaped bodies and cestodes have bodies composed of segments or proglottids.

Flukes. Flukes, or trematodes, are flatworms that have leaf-shaped bodies. Most are hermaphroditic, with male and female sex organs in a single body. Their digestive systems are incomplete and consist of only sack-like tubes. Their life cycle is complex; snails serve as first intermediate hosts and other aquatic animals or plants serve as second intermediate hosts.

Examples of flukes include the sheep liver fluke, *Fasciola hepatica*, the intestinal fluke, *Fasciolopsis buski*, and the blood fluke, *Schistosoma* spp.

Free-living amebae. Amebae that are present in soil or in warm freshwater ponds or swimming pools and can be opportunistic pathogens, causing meningoencephalitis or keratitis. See *Acanthamoeba*, *Balamuthia mandrillaris*, and *Naegleria fowleri*.

Gambian sleeping sickness. A form of African trypanosomiasis due to the hemoflagellate *Trypanosoma brucei gambiense*. The infection is transmitted by the bite of the tsetse fly and is limited to tropical West and Central Africa. The incubation period varies from a few days to weeks. *T. brucei gambiense* produces chronic disease that often ends fatally, with central nervous system (CNS) involvement after several years' duration. The organisms invade the lymph nodes and produce fever, myalgia, arthralgia, and lymphadenopathy. Chronic disease progresses to CNS involvement with lethargy, tremors, and general deterioration. Ultimately, seizures, hemiplegia, and incontinence occur and the patient becomes comatose. Death results from CNS damage and concomitant infections, such as pneumonia and malaria.

Giardia lamblia (*duodenalis*). An intestinal flagellate that exists in both a motile trophozoite stage and a cyst stage. Infection is acquired by ingestion of contaminated food and water as well as by human-to-human spread via the fecal-oral or oral-anal route. G. lamblia parasitizes the proximal small bowel, resulting in either asymptomatic carriage or symptomatic disease ranging from a mild diarrhea to a severe malabsorption syndrome. The onset of disease is sudden and consists of foul-smelling, watery diarrhea, abdominal cramps, flatulence, and steatorrhea. Blood and pus are rarely present in the stool. Diagnosis is made by detecting the characteristic cysts and trophozoites in stool and duodenal aspirates examined microscopically. Both immunofluorescent stains and antigen detection assays are also available (1).

Ground itch. See Creeping eruption.

Helminths. Complex multicellular organisms (worms) that are elongated and bilaterally symmetrical. The helminths include nematodes (roundworms), trematodes (flukes), and cestodes (tapeworms) and, in general, are macroscopic, ranging in size from 1 mm to 1 meter or more.

Hookworm. The two hookworms in humans are *Ancylostoma duodenale* (Old World hookworm) and *Necator americanus* (New World hookworm). The hookworm life cycle begins with a filariform larva which penetrates the skin, enters the circulation, and migrates to the lungs, where it is coughed up and then swallowed, and finally develops to adulthood in the small intestine. Both species have mouthparts designed for sucking blood from injured intestinal tissue. Adult worms produce nausea, vomiting, and diarrhea. Daily blood loss is estimated at 0.15 to 0.25 ml for each adult *A. duodenale* and 0.03 ml for each adult *N. americanus* that parasitizes the small bowel. Over time, and depending on the worm burden, a microcytic hypochromic (iron deficiency) anemia develops due to the chronic blood loss. Hookworm infections occur primarily in tropical and subtropical areas and in the southern United States.

Hydatid cysts. See *Echinococcus.*

Hymenolepis nana. Also known as the dwarf tape-worm, *H. nana* is only 2 to 4 cm in length. Infection is initiated when embryonated eggs are ingested and develop in the intestine into a larval cysticercoid stage. The cysticercoid larva attaches to the small intestine via its four muscular suckers and crown of hooklets and, on maturation, produces a strobila of egg-laden proglottids. The eggs passing in the feces are immediately infective, creating the potential of auto-infection, which can lead to a very heavy worm burden and severe clinical symptoms of diarrhea, abdominal pain, and anorexia. Diagnosis is made by microscopic examination of stool, which reveals the characteristic egg with its six-hooked embryo and polar filaments.

Isospora belli. A unicellular coccidian parasite of the intestinal epithelium. Both sexual and asexual reproduction may occur in the intestine. The oocyst is the diagnostic stage detected in fecal specimens. Infection may produce mild to severe gastrointestinal disease that mimics the malabsorption syndrome seen with giardiasis. *Isopora* infection in individuals with AIDS is often associated with chronic diarrhea, weight loss, anorexia, malaise, and fatigue. Infection with this organism follows ingestion of contaminated food or water or oral-anal sexual contact.

Kala-azar. See Dumdum fever.

Katayama's syndrome. Seen in schistosomiasis, Katayama's syndrome occurs at the onset of oviposition by the adult worm and is marked by fever, chills, cough, urticaria, arthralgias, lymphadenopathy, splenomegaly, and abdominal pain. Typically developing 1 to 2 months after primary exposure to schistosome larvae, this syndrome may persist for 3 months or more. It is thought to be a reaction to a massive release of parasite antigens that triggers immune complex formation. Laboratory findings include leukocytosis, eosinophilia, and polyclonal gammopathy.

Kinetoplast. An accessory organelle found in many protozoa, especially the trypanosomes. The kinetoplast consists of a large mitochondrion next to the blepharoplast (basal body origin of the flagella) of the anterior or undulating membrane flagellum. The kinetoplast contains mitochondrial DNA.

Larva. An immature stage in the development of a worm before it becomes a mature adult. Roundworms (nematodes) molt several times during their development, and each subsequent larval stage is increasingly more mature.

***Leishman-Donovan* bodies.** The small ovoid amastigote forms observed within the tissue macrophages of the liver and spleen in patients with *Leishmania donovani* infection.

Leishmania. Flagellated, insect-transmitted protozoa that infect blood and tissues. Three species of *Leishmania* produce disease in humans: *L. donovani, L. tropica*, and *L. braziliensis*. The diseases caused by these species are distinguished by the ability of the organism to infect deep tissues (visceral leishmaniasis; *L. donovani*), cutaneous (*L. tropica*), or mucocutaneous (*L. braziliensis*) tissues. All forms of leishmaniasis are transmitted by sandflies.

Liver flukes. Trematodes that parasitize the bile ducts of humans and animals. The two medically significant liver flukes are *Fasciola hepatica* and *Opisthorchis* (*Clonorchis*) *sinensis*.

Loa loa. Also known as the African eyeworm, *Loa loa* is an agent of filariasis. The adult worms can migrate through subcutaneous tissues, muscle, and characteristically in front of the eyeball. The migration of the adult worms produces calabar swellings. *L. loa* infection is transmitted by the bite of a fly called *Crysops*. Microfilariae are produced about 6 months after the initial infection and can persist for years. The sheathed microfilariae may be detected in the blood and are present during daytime hours. *L. loa* is confined to the equatorial rain forests of Africa.

Malaria. A disease caused by one of four species of *Plasmodium*: *P. falciparum*, *P. vivax*, *P. malariae*, and *P. ovale*. The plasmodia are protozoan parasites of red blood cells and are transmitted by mosquitoes. Malaria is a disease marked by periodic high-spiking fevers, chills, and rigors. The intensity of clinical signs and symptoms varies with the species of *Plasmodium* and the degree of parasitemia. Infection due to *P. falciparum* is the most severe and may be life-threatening, especially among young children and other nonimmune individuals. Infection with the other species is milder but may be chronic and relapsing (*P. vivax* and *P. ovale*). Hemolysis caused by the infecting parasite may result in anemia and renal failure (9).

Malayan filariasis. See *Brugia malayi* and Filariasis.

Mansonella. Filarial nematodes including *M. perstans*, *M. streptocerca*, and *M. ozzardi*. Infections due to *Mansonella* species are generally asymptomatic but may cause dermatitis, lymphadenitis, hydrocele, and, rarely, lymphatic obstruction leading to elephantiasis. All the *Mansonella* species produce nonsheathed microfilariae and are transmitted by biting midges or black flies. The microfilariae may be detected by examination of blood films. See also Filariasis.

Maurer's dots. Reddish granules or clefts that may be observed in Giemsa-stained erythrocytes parasitized by *Plasmodium falciparum*.

Metazoa. A subkingdom of animals consisting of all multicellular organisms in which cells are differentiated to form tissue. Includes all animals except protozoa.

Microfilaria. A term used for the larval form of a filarial worm, usually in the blood or tissues of a human host. Microfilariae are ingested by the arthropod intermediate host.

Microfilariasis. See Filariasis.

Microspora. A phylum consisting of small intra-cellular parasites (the microsporidia) that are charac-terized by the structure of their spores, which have a complex tubular extrusion mechanism (polar tubule) used to inject the infective material (sporoplasm) into host cells. These organisms were formerly classified with the Sporozoa (2).

Microsporidia. Obligate intracellular pathogens belonging to the phylum Microspora. Microsporidia lack mitochondria, peroxisomes, Golgi, and other typical eukaryotic organelles. Microsporidia have been detected in human tissues and implicated as participants in disease in humans. To date, six genera of microsporidia (*Encephalitozoon, Pleistophora, Nosema, Vittaforma, Trachipleistophora,* and *Enterocytozoon*) and unclassified *Microsporidium* species have been reported in humans (2).

Miracidium. Ciliated first-stage, free-swimming larva of a trematode (fluke), which emerges from an egg and must penetrate the appropriate species of snail to continue its life cycle.

Naegleria fowleri. See Free-living amebae. *N. fowleri* is the most common cause of acute primary amebic meningoencephalitis. In *Naegleria* infection only trophozoites, no cysts, are observed in tissue. This organism lives in freshwater and causes infection by colonization of the nasal passages with subsequent invasion of the nasal mucosa and extension into the brain. Destruction of brain tissue, usually the frontal lobes, is characterized by a fulminant, rapidly fatal meningoencephalitis.

Necator americanus. See Hookworm. *N. americanus* is known as the New World hookworm. It differs from *Ancylostoma duodenale* (Old World hookworm) in geographic distribution, size (*N. americanus* is smaller), and structure of mouthparts (chitinous plates [*N. americanus*] versus chitinous teeth [*A. duodenale*]).

Nematode. Members of the phylum Nematoda, which consists of the roundworms, characterized by a cylindrical body. The sexes of roundworms are separate, and these organisms have a complete digestive system. The nematodes include blood and tissue parasites, as well as intestinal parasites.

Nosema. An obligate intracellular parasite belonging to the phylum *Microspora*. *Nosema* has been reported to cause keratitis, myositis, and disseminated infections in immunocompromised individuals. *N. connori* has been observed to cause infection involving the muscles of the stomach, bowel, arteries, diaphragm, and heart, with additional dissemination to the liver, lungs, and adrenal glands. See Microsporidia (2).

Onchocerca volvulus. A filarial nematode that is endemic in many parts of Africa. Following the bite of the black fly (*Simulium*) vector, the larvae migrate to the subcutaneous tissues and develop into adult worms. The adults become encased in fibrous tissue and may remain viable for as many as 15 years. Production of nonsheathed microfilariae results in clinical manifestations of onchocerciasis as the microfilariae migrate to the skin, eyes, and other tissues. The clinical signs and symptoms are the result of both acute and chronic inflammatory reaction to microfilarial antigens. Involvement of the eyes often leads to blindness (river blindness) and a number of skin conditions, including pruritis, hyperkeratosis, and myxedematous thickening, are related to the presence of this parasite.

Operculum. The lid- or cap-like cover on certain helminth (worm) eggs.

Opisthorchis sinensis. Formerly known as *Clonorchis sinensis*, the Chinese liver fluke. *O. sinensis* is found in China, Japan, Korea, and Vietnam. Its life cycle involves two intermediate hosts, a snail and freshwater fish. The cercariae encyst in the tissue of the fish and then infect humans when uncooked fish containing the metacercariae are eaten. The flukes develop first in the duodenum and then migrate to the bile ducts, where they mature into adults. Eggs produced by the mature flukes are passed with feces and are subsequently eaten by snails. Infection is usually asymptomatic; however, severe infection with many worms may lead to biliary obstruction. Chronic infection with accompanying inflammation may lead to adenocarcinoma of the biliary tree.

Oriental blood fluke. See *Schistosoma japonicum.*

Oriental sore. See Delhi boil.

Paragonimus westermani. Commonly called the lung fluke, *P. westermani* causes infection (paragonimiasis) in many countries in Asia, Africa, India, and Latin America. It has a typical fluke life cycle involving both a snail and a freshwater crustacean (crabs and crayfish) intermediate host. Humans become infected when they consume infected meat. The larvae excyst in the stomach, migrate through the intestinal wall and the abdominal cavity, and finally penetrate the diaphragm to ultimately reside in the lungs. Clinical symptoms may reflect the inflammation associated with the larval migration or from adults residing in the lungs or other ectopic tissues. Fever, cough, production of blood-tinged sputum, and chest pain may progress to dyspnea, chronic bronchitis, and pleural effusions. Eggs may be detected in the sputum. Migration of the larvae to the central nervous system produces severe neurologic disease (visual defects, seizures, motor weakness) referred to as cerebral paragonimiasis.

Parasites. Organisms that live on or in another organism and that have a metabolic dependence on the larger host species. Parasites are complex eukaryotic microbes that may be either unicellular or multicellular. They range in size from protozoa as small as 1 to 2 μm in diameter to arthropods and tapeworms that can measure up to 10 m in length.

Pinworm. See *Enterobius vermicularis.*

Plasmodium. See Malaria.

Platyhelminthes. Phylum Platyhelminthes consists of the flatworms, which have flattened bodies that are leaf-like or resemble ribbon segments. Platyhelminthes can be further divided into trematodes (flukes) and cestodes (tapeworms). See Flatworms, Flukes, and Cestodes.

Pork tapeworm. See *Taenia* and Cysticercosis.

Protozoa. Unicellular eukaryotic organisms including amebae, flagellates, ciliates, and coccidia.

Pseudopod. A protoplasmic extension (false-foot) of the trophozoites of amebae that allows them to move and to engulf food.

Pumpkinseed tapeworm. See *Dipylidium caninum*.

River blindness. Refers to blindness caused by migrating microfilariae of *Onchocerca volvulus*.

Romana's sign. Classic periorbital edema secondary to the bite of a triatomid bug (vector of Chagas' disease).

Roundworms. See Nematode.

Sarcocystis lindemanni. A coccidian parasite closely related to *Isospora belli* and *Toxoplasma gondii*. *S. lindemanni* occurs worldwide as a parasite of sheep, cattle, and pigs. Infection in humans may occur following the ingestion of infected raw or under-cooked meat. Most infections are asymptomatic, but myositis and eosinophilia may occur on rare occasions.

Schistosoma. Trematodes (flukes) that differ from other flukes in that they have cylindrical bodies and separate male and female forms. The schistosomes are also known as blood flukes, referring to the fact that they are obligate intravascular parasites. The adult flukes are not found in cavities, ducts, or other tissues. The three schistosomes most frequently associated with human disease are *S. mansoni*, *S. haematobium*, and *S. japonicum*. All schistosomes have life cycles that involve freshwater snails. Following development in a snail, the infective free-swimming cercariae penetrate intact skin, enter the circulation, and develop in the intracellular portal circulation (*S. mansoni* and *S. japonicum*) or the vesicle, prostatic, rectal, and uterine venous plexuses (*S. haematobium*). The adult worms may persist within the vasculature for 20 to 30 years, during which time they mate and produce eggs that pass through the tissue into the lumen of the bowel and bladder. Although there is little host reaction to the adult worms, the eggs elicit an intense inflammatory response that results in tissue destruction, microabscesses, and eventually fibrosis and scarring. The eggs may be retained in tissues where they cause granuloma formation and fibrosis, the clinical significance of which depends on the anatomic location and the number of eggs. Also see Katayama's syndrome.

Schizogony. Asexual multiplication of sporozoan (coccidian) parasites. Multiple intracellular nuclear divisions preceding cytoplasmic division. See also Coccidia.

Schüffner's dots. Dot-like densities in erythrocytes infected with *Plasmodium vivax*. Seen best in blood films stained with Giemsa stain.

Septata. See *Encephalitozoon* and Microsporidia (2).

Sheep liver fluke. See *Fasciola hepatica*.

Sleeping sickness. A form of African trypanosomiasis due to central nervous system involvement with *Trypanosoma brucei gambiense* and *Trypanosoma brucei rhodesiense*. See also Gambian sleeping sickness and *Trypanosoma*.

Snail fever. An alternative/common name referring to schistosomiasis. See Bilharziasis, Katayama's syndrome, and *Schistosoma*.

Sporogony. Sexual reproduction of sporozoan (coccidian) parasites. Production of spores and sporozoites. See also Coccidia.

String test. Technique used for the diagnosis of infection due to *Giardia lamblia*. Marketed as the Entero-Test (HDC Corp., San Jose, Calif.), this test consists of a weighted capsule containing gelatin and a tightly wound string. One end of the string is taped to the patient's cheek and the capsule is swallowed, allowing the remainder of the string to enter the duodenum and proximal ileum. After approximately 5 h the string is removed from the patient and the adherent material (mucus, etc.) is examined microscopically as a wet mount or permanent stained smear.

Strongyloides stercoralis. An intestinal nematode found in the small bowel, *S. stercoralis* may exist free-living in soil where rhabditiform larvae are produced. The rhabditiform larvae may either continue the free-living cycle or develop into infective filariform larvae that penetrate intact skin and migrate via the circulation to the lungs where they are coughed up, swallowed, and then develop into adults in the small intestine. The adult worm produces about one dozen eggs per day. The eggs usually hatch within the mucosa of the bowel and the rhabditiform larvae are passed in the stool. In autoinfection the rhabditiform larvae do not pass in the feces but develop into filariform larvae within the bowel and initiate the infection cycle. Most infections are asymptomatic, but heavy worm loads may cause peptic ulcer-like symptoms, and the hyperinfection syndrome caused by massive autoinfection may be fatal. Diagnosis is made by detection of larvae in the stool.

Swimmer's itch. See Cercarial dermatitis.

Taenia. The genus *Taenia* encompasses two tape-worms that may cause infection in humans, *T. solium* (also see Cysticercosis) and *T. saginata. T. solium* is also known as the pork tapeworm. The larvae of *T. solium* encyst in pork muscle (see Cysticercus or Bladder worm) and, on ingestion by a human host, the larval scolex attaches to the wall of the small bowel. The worm then produces proglottids until a chain or strobila of proglottids, which may be several meters long, is developed. The mature proglottids contain eggs and are passed in the feces. The eggs are ingested by pigs, hatch in the pig intestine, and penetrate the wall where the larvae enter the circulation and migrate to the tissues. In humans, ingestion of the eggs results in cysticercosis.

T. saginata is also known as the beef tapeworm. The life cycle of *T. saginata* is similar to that of *T. solium*, except that the tissue phase takes place in beef cattle.

Once infected beef is ingested, the worm develops in the small intestine where it may attain a length of up to 10 m. Although it is possible for humans to ingest the eggs, cysticercosis produced by *T. saginata* does not occur in humans.

Clinical signs and symptoms of intestinal infection with either of the *Taenia* species are usually absent, but vague abdominal pains and chronic indigestion have been reported. The eggs of *T. saginata* and *T. solium* are indistinguishable, but the species may be differentiated by the morphology of the proglottids and scolex.

Tapeworms. See Cestodes.

Toxocara. The genus *Toxocara* includes the ascarid worms *T. canis* and *T. cati*, which are normally found in the intestines of dogs and cats, respectively. Infection in humans is accidental and produces a disease known as visceral larva migrans or toxocariasis. When the eggs are ingested by humans, the resulting larval forms are unable to develop normally and may migrate to extraintestinal sites where they eventually die. The clinical manifestations of toxocariasis are related to the migration of the larvae through the tissues and the accompanying host response. The migrating larvae can induce bleeding, eosinophilia, and necrosis. Signs and symptoms are related to the overall worm burden and the organs involved. The organs most commonly involved include the lungs, heart, kidneys, liver, skeletal muscles, eyes, and central nervous system. Diagnosis is based on clinical findings, the presence of eosinophilia, known exposure to dogs or cats, and serologic confirmation. Examination of the feces from infected patients is not helpful, because the egg-laying adult worms are not present.

Toxoplasma gondii. A coccidian parasite related to *Plasmodium*, *Isospora*, and other members of the phylum Apicomplexa. *T. gondii* is an intracellular parasite of humans and a wide variety of animals. The reservoir host is the common house cat. Organisms develop in the intestinal cells of the cat and are passed in feces, where they mature into infective cysts in the external environment. When ingested, the oocysts can produce acute and chronic infection of various tissues, including the brain. Humans become infected in either of two ways: (i) ingestion of infective oocysts from contaminated cat feces and (ii) ingestion of improperly cooked meat from animals that serve as intermediate hosts (usually beef).

Trematodes. See Flukes.

Trichinella spiralis. A nematode that is the etiologic agent of trichinosis. The adult worm lives in the duodenal and jejunal mucosa of the flesh-eating mammals worldwide. The infectious larval form is encysted in striated muscle tissue of carnivorous and omnivorous animals. The life cycle is simple and direct. Ingestion of infected meat releases the larvae, which then develop into adult worms within the small intestine. The female worm produces infective larvae, which then penetrate the intestinal mucosa and gain access to the circulation where they are carried to various muscle sites. In humans the larvae encyst in the muscle and eventually die and calcify. Clinical symptoms are related to the worm burden and the location of the larval cysts. The muscles invaded most commonly are the extraocular muscles of the eye, the tongue, the deltoid, pectoral, and intracostal muscles, the diaphragm, and the gastrocnemius muscle.

Trichomonas. A genus of flagellate protozoan that includes both pathogenic (*T. vaginalis*) and non-pathogenic (*T. tenax* [oral], *T. hominis* [intestinal]) species. *T. vaginalis* is a cause of genitourinary tract infections. *T. vaginalis* exists only as a trophozoite and is characterized by four flagellae and a short undulating membrane. It has a characteristic jerking motility that may be observed on a wet mount of vaginal secretions. Infection with *T. vaginalis* is transmitted by sexual intercourse and involves the urethra and vagina of women and prostate gland of men. Vaginitis and urethritis are associated with itching, burning, and painful urination. Men are primarily carriers but may experience urethritis and/or prostatitis.

Trichuris trichiura. An intestinal nematode commonly known as whipworm. The life cycle is simple, with ingested eggs hatching in the small intestine and migration of the larval worm to the cecum. The worms mature to adults in the cecum and produce eggs at a rate of 3,000 to 10,000 per day. Eggs passed in the stool mature in soil and become infectious in 3 weeks. The eggs of *T. trichiura* are distinctive, with a barrel shape and the presence of polar plugs at each end of the egg. Clinical manifestations are related to the intensity of the worm burden. Large numbers of worms may produce abdominal pain and distention. Prolapse of the rectum may be seen as a result of the irritation and straining during defecation. Anemia and eosinophilia may be seen in severe infections.

Trophozoite. The motile stage of a protozoan which feeds, multiplies, and maintains the presence of the organism within the host.

Trypanosoma. A genus of hemoflagellates that includes the agents of African trypanosomiasis, or sleeping sickness (*T. brucei gambiense* and *T. brucei rhodesiense*), and the agent of American trypanosomiasis, or Chagas' disease (*T. cruzi*). The agents of

African trypanosomiasis are transmitted by tsetse flies and cause central nervous system infection. *T. brucei rhodesiense* is found in East Africa and causes a more severe form of sleeping sickness that progresses rapidly into fatal illness. This organism is more virulent than *T. brucei gambiense* and develops in greater numbers in the blood. Lymphadenopathy is uncommon and CNS invasion occurs early with accompanying lethargy, anorexia, and mental disturbance. Infected people are usually dead in 9 to 12 months if their disease is untreated. See also Gambian sleeping sickness and Chagas' disease.

Trypomastigote. A developmental form of hemoflagellate with the kinetoplast located posteriorly and an undulating membrane that extends along the entire body from the flagellum (anterior end) to the posterior end at the blepharoplast. This form is seen in the blood of humans with trypanosomiasis and as the infective stage in the insect vector.

Wuchereria bancrofti. The agent of Bancroft's filariasis, *W. bancrofti* is a filarial nematode that parasitizes the lymphatic system of infected individuals in Central Africa, Asia, and the Mediterranean. The sheathed microfilaria circulate in the blood with a nocturnal periodicity and may be detected in Giemsa-stained blood films. As with *Brugia malayi,* *W. bancrofti* causes lymphedema that leads to elephantiasis. See also Bancroft's filariasis, *Brugia malayi*, Elephantiasis, and Filariasis.

Xenodiagnosis. Infections with *Trypanosoma cruzi* may be diagnosed by allowing an uninfected *Triatoma* bug to feed on the patient; the insect's feces are later examined for parasites (trypanosome forms).

REFERENCES

1. **Adam, R. D.** 2001. Biology of *Giardia lamblia*. *Clin. Microbiol. Rev.* **14:**447–475.

2. **Franzen, C., and A. Müller.** 1999. Molecular techniques for detection, species differentiation, and phylogenetic analysis of microsporidia. *Clin. Microbiol. Rev.* **12:**243–285.

3. **Garcia, L. S.** 2001. *Diagnostic Medical Parasitology*, 4th ed. ASM Press, Washington, D.C.

4. **Homer, M. J., I. Aguilar-Delfin, S. R. Telford III, P. J. Krause, and D. H. Persing.** 2000. Babesiosis. *Clin. Microbiol. Rev.* **13:**451–469.

5. **Hunter, P. R., and G. Nichols.** 2002. Epidemiology and clinical features of *Cryptosporidium* infection in immunocompromised patients. *Clin. Microbiol. Rev.* **15:**145–154.

6. **Murray, P. R., G. S. Kobayashi, M. A. Pfaller, and K. S. Rosenthal.** 2002. *Medical Microbiology*, 4th ed. Mosby, St. Louis, Mo.

7. **Murray, P. R., E. J. Baron, J. H. Jorgensen, M. A. Pfaller, and R. H. Yolken.** 2003. *Manual of Clinical Microbiology*, 8th ed. ASM Press, Washington, D.C.

8. **Pfaller, M. A.** 2002. Parasitology, p. 1291–1344. *In* K. D. McClatchey (ed.), *Clinical Laboratory Medicine*, 2nd ed. Lippincott Williams & Wilkins, Philadelphia, Pa.

9. **Phillips, R. S.** 2001. Current status of malaria and potential for control. *Clin. Microbiol. Rev.* **14:**206–226.

10. **Stenzel, D. J., and P. F. BoreLanz.** 1996. *Blastocystis hominis* revisited. *Clin. Microbiol. Rev.* **9:**563–584.

Viruses

Adenoviruses. A large group of DNA viruses numbered variously from 1 through 51. Viruses of this group are numbered rather than given specific names. Adenoviruses can cause a variety of upper and lower respiratory tract infections (common cold, pharyngitis, tonsillitis; types 1 to 7), epidemic respiratory tract infection among military recruits, epidemic keratoconjunctivitis (types 8 and 37), acute hemorrhagic cystitis (types 11 and 21), and diarrhea (types 2, 31, 40, and 41). Occasionally, adenovirus infection can be severe and generalized. These infections may be transmitted from person to person by respiratory droplets or by the fecal-oral route.

Alphaviruses. These togaviruses are RNA viruses that represent important agents of viral, mosquito-borne encephalitis in humans, horses, and birds.

These include Eastern, Western, and Venezuelan equine encephalitis.

Arboviruses. A heterogeneous group of more than 150 arthropod-borne viruses that cause infections in humans, including related zoonotic viruses such as hantaviruses. Most infections result in nonspecific febrile illnesses. However, some arboviral infections cause sudden-onset, severe headache, myalgia, and lumbar pain. The most prominent members of the arbovirus group include hantaviruses, California encephalitis, Colorado tick fever, dengue, Ebola, Japanese encephalitis, LaCrosse, Eastern equine encephalitis (EEE), Venezuelan equine encephalitis (VEE), Western equine encephalitis (WEE), St. Louis encephalitis, Lassa fever, Marburg, Rift Valley fever, vesicular stomatitis, West Nile, and yellow fever.

Arenaviruses. A small group of six RNA viruses that cause viral hemorrhagic fevers in humans. They are rare in the United States, but important in Africa and South America. Most prominent in this group are lymphotropic choriomeningitis virus and Lassa fever virus. Lymphotropic choriomeningitis virus can be relatively mild, and causes fever, myalgia, headache, and weakness. However, meningitis and encephalitis can ensue; birth defects can occur during in utero infection. Lassa fever virus is much more severe, with disease progressing over a period of 2 weeks and culminating with hepatic, myocardial, and pulmonary damage, with or without obvious hemorrhages, that results in death in 15 to 20% of patients. Both viruses occur naturally in rodents and appear to be transmitted through the urine and feces of the rodents to humans.

Astroviruses. The eight serotypes of astroviruses primarily cause gastrointestinal infections characterized by vomiting, abdominal pain, diarrhea, and fever. They occur most frequently in young children (20).

B-19 virus. See Parvovirus B-19.

Betavirus. A herpesvirus. See Cytomegalovirus.

BK virus. A widely distributed virus that causes primarily asymptomatic infections; it can remain latent in the kidney. However, viral latency may result in reactivation during later periods of cellular immune dysfunction, leading to severe and even fatal disseminated disease. The virus is thought to be transmitted primarily by inhalation of respiratory droplets, although other routes, including exposure to infected blood or body fluids, cannot be excluded (3).

Bunyaviruses. A group of Arboviruses that are spread directly to humans by contact with rodent urine or feces. Most notably, hantavirus causes a hemorrhagic fever with diffuse capillary dysfunction (35).

Caliciviruses. These RNA viruses include the gastroenteritis group (primarily Norwalk) and the hepatitis group (hepatitis E).

Colorado tick fever. Characterized by rash, nausea, vomiting, and high fever. It is caused by a coltivirus of the family *Reoviridae*. Humans, predominantly in the western United States, are infected by the bite of a tick that has fed on an infected squirrel or chipmunk.

Coltivirus. See Colorado tick fever.

Coronavirus. A group of RNA viruses most often associated with the common cold or with diarrhea. However, a newly described coronavirus has been named as the putative agent of the severe acute respiratory syndrome (SARS; see also SARS, below) (26).

Coxsackie viruses. Coxsackie A and B can cause aseptic meningitis and are transmitted by the fecal-oral route. Coxsackie A can cause a vesicular rash on hands and feet and oral-pharyngeal lesions (hand-foot-mouth disease). Coxsackie B can cause pleuritic chest pain, pancreatitis, and, most significantly, myocarditis.

Creutzfeldt-Jakob disease (CJD). A severe, transmissible neurologic syndrome possibly caused by a prion. It is a rare cause of dementia that occurs sporadically by unknown means of transmission. However, iatrogenic cases of CJD (iCJD) have occurred in certain transplant recipients, laboratory workers, and surgeons who had direct contact with infected tissues or contaminated surgical instruments (17). A variant of CJD (vCJD) in humans has been associated with consumption of meat products contaminated with the bovine spongiform encephalopathy agent (BSE), especially in the United Kingdom (16).

Cytomegalovirus (CMV). An important cause of congenital, perinatal, and postnatal infections throughout the world. It is often asymptomatic, or it may cause an mononucleosis-like infection in young adults (less common than Epstein-Barr virus), but it can cause retinitis, pneumonia, myocarditis, and hepatitis in immunosuppressed patients, such as those receiving cancer chemotherapy or organ transplants, or patients with AIDS. Transmission can occur transplacentally, at birth, through sexual contact, or through contact with contaminated blood or body fluids. Reactivation of latent CMV infection can occur during immunosuppression.

Dane particle. Old name for hepatitis B virus.

Dengue fever viruses. A group of flaviviruses transmitted by mosquitoes in many tropical areas that cause high fever, nausea, rash, and bone pain. Dengue hemorrhagic fever is characterized by hypotension, shock, and gastrointestinal bleeding.

Dependovirus. An adenovirus-dependent covirus infection.

Eastern equine encephalitis virus. See Alphaviruses.

Ebola. See Filoviruses.

Echo viruses. Include many different types that can commonly cause diarrhea and aseptic meningitis. They may also cause disseminated neonatal infection, including hepatitis, and encephalitis.

Enteroviruses. Refers to a genus of viruses, including coxsackie, echo, hepatitis A, and polio, and to numbered viruses that correspond to species, e.g., enterovirus 70 (acute conjunctivitis), or enterovirus 71 (encephalitis). The majority of infections are asymptomatic or represent an acute nonspecific febrile illness (resembling a common cold) with or without a rash. However, meningitis due to enteroviruses represent an important cause of hospitalization of many young children (34).

Epstein-Barr virus (EBV). The most common cause of infectious mononucleosis in young adults. It is characterized by fever, malaise, pharyngitis, lymphadenopathy, and lymphocytosis. However, it is also associated with several lymphoproliferative disorders (LPDs) in immunocompromised patients, including oral hairy leukoplakia in patients with AIDS. In nonimmunosuppressed patients, EBV is associated with Burkitt's lymphoma, nasopharyngeal carcinoma, Hodgkin's disease, gastric adenocarcinoma, and several less common carcinomas (21). It is transmitted through oral contact (saliva), and perhaps by sexual contact.

Flaviviruses. A group of RNA viruses that include the mosquito-borne epidemic viruses (dengue, Japanese encephalitis, St. Louis encephalitis, and yellow fever), as well as hepatitis C virus.

Filoviruses. RNA viruses that cause severe and highly communicable hemorrhagic fevers, including Ebola and Marburg viruses. Both diseases are characterized by sudden onset of fever, chills, pharyngitis, headache, myalgia, and anorexia, followed later by nausea, vomiting, abdominal pain, and diarrhea. After a few days, a maculopapular rash develops over the trunk. The rash becomes petechial and hemorrhagic, and mucous membrane and gastrointestinal hemorrhages occur. Coagulation problems, including disseminated intravascular coagulation, and multi-organ failure often result in death. Both viruses appear to have various monkeys as the natural host. Most infections have been acquired in Africa or by contact with monkeys or their tissues emanating from Africa (23).

Gammavirus. See Herpesviruses.

Hantavirus. The causative agent of hantavirus pulmonary syndrome. A virus that causes zoonotic infections when humans are exposed to aerosols derived from the urine and feces of mice.

Hepadnaviruses. Double-stranded DNA viruses that include hepatitis B ("Dane particle").

Hepatitis viruses. A group of genetically unrelated viruses that share only the characteristic of infecting the liver and causing hepatitis. See Caliciviruses, Hepadnaviruses, and Picornaviruses.

> **Hepatitis A (HAV).** A picornavirus of the enterovirus group. It causes acute, usually self-limited hepatitis following acquisition by the fecal-oral route. It is estimated to represent 20 to 25% of viral hepatitis cases worldwide. Hepatitis A has often occurred as outbreaks related to contaminated food or water, or to consumption of

contaminated shellfish. There is now an effective vaccine that can prevent HAV (40).

Hepatitis B virus (HBV; "Dane particle"). HBV is an enveloped DNA virus that is a highly important cause of asymptomatic, acute, or chronic hepatitis ("serum hepatitis"). It is transmitted by transfusion or percutaneous injury with contaminated blood, by needle sharing, through transplantation of infected organs, by sexual contact, and at birth or through breast-feeding to newborns (29). Different antigens of the HBV structure are used for laboratory diagnosis and disease classification.

Hepatitis C (HCV). An RNA virus of the flavivirus group that has been referred to as the agent of non-A, non-B, or "post-transfusion" hepatitis. It causes asymptomatic, acute, or chronic hepatitis, and occasionally leads to hepatocellular carcinoma. It is a much more common cause of hepatitis than originally appreciated. It is acquired by needle sharing, transfusion with contaminated blood, contamination during hemodialysis, organ transplantation, and, less frequently, sexual contact (1).

Hepatitis D ("Delta agent"). An RNA virus that is by itself "defective" in lacking an essential outer envelope that it can only acquire from coinfection or as a superinfection with HBV (37). It most commonly occurs among injection-drug users or others at high risk of HBV infection. It can convert a mild or chronic HBV infection into a fulminant, rapidly progressive disease.

Hepatitis E (HEV). An RNA virus of the calicivirus group. It causes acute hepatitis without major sequelae in most patients or a carrier state. However, there is a high rate of fulminant hepatitis in pregnant females in their third trimester. It is transmitted by the fecal-oral route, principally by contaminated water in developing countries, perhaps contaminated by wild animals with HEV infection (38).

Hepatitis G (HGV). HGV is related to HCV, but its exact clinical significance remains to be fully elucidated. It has been demonstrated to be transmitted by blood transfusion (2). Of note, coinfection with HGV appears to improve survival of patients with HIV infection.

Herpesviruses. A family of double-stranded DNA viruses that includes alpha-, beta-, and gammaviruses.

Alphaviruses.

Herpes simplex virus 1 (HSV-1). Causes gingivostomatitis or cold sores (herpes labialis), pharyngitis, vesicular finger lesions (herpes whitlow), conjunctivitis or keratitis (common), and, occasionally, severe encephalitis. Herpes is the most common cause of fatal, sporadic encephalitis in the United States. Latency and recurrences are common due to persistence of the virus in various dorsal root ganglia (39).

Herpes simplex virus 2 (HSV-2). Causes relapsing, painful vesicular genital lesions after sexual contact, herpes whitlow, occasionally meningitis in adults, and neonatal encephalitis from an infected mother (15).

Herpes B virus. Also called herpesvirus simiae, is an important zoonotic infection that can be transmitted by Old World monkeys (especially macaques) to humans. In humans it causes a severe, often fatal neurologic disease with encephalitis (7).

Varicella-zoster virus (VZV). See Varicella-zoster virus, below.

Betavirus. See Cytomegalovirus.

Gammavirus. See Epstein-Barr virus and human herpesvirus-6.

Human herpesvirus 6, 7, and 8 (HHV-6, -7, and -8).

HHV-6. Now known as HHV-6A and -6B. HHV-6 causes roseola or sixth disease (rose-colored rash with fever; most often due to HHV-6B) in children who are usually less than 2 years of age. The rash usually starts on the neck and back, then the extremities, with the face spared. The fever may result in seizures in some children. Transmission is by saliva or other respiratory droplets. Immuno-suppressed children or adults can have rash-associated illness from virus reactivation, which may disseminate in some individuals. In addition, HHV-6 has been speculated to be involved in AIDS progression and in various lymphoproliferative diseases; it has even been cited as a possible cause of multiple sclerosis (5).

HHV-7. Responsible for only about 10% of roseola cases, and may result in a milder infection. Like HHV-6, it can be latent in lymphocytes and can cause reactivation infections in immunosup-pressed patients, often in conjunction with CMV infection.

HHV-8. Occurs frequently in Africa, but much less so in the United States and Europe. Primary HHV-8 infections may be mild and unapparent, probably being acquired early in childhood through contact with saliva. However, there is some evidence for sexual transmission in adults, in particular in men who have sex with men. In that setting, HHV-8 is best known for its association with Kaposi's sarcoma (KS) (11). There are several varieties of KS, but all are characterized by a reddish-brown plaque or nodular lesions on the trunk, extremities, or oral cavity. In addition, HHV-8 has been associated with a group of aggressive lymphomas known as primary effusion lymphomas (PELs), with multicentric Castleman's disease (MCD), and with several other lympho-proliferative disorders.

HIV. Human immunodeficiency viruses 1 and 2. Acute HIV infection (acute retroviral syndrome) of HIV-1 presents initially with fever and rash, and often lymphadenopathy. Progressive infection of the CD4 lymphocytes leads to their progressive decrease in number and resulting loss of T-cell-mediated immunity. When CD4 cells drop to very low levels (usually <200 per μl), the acquired immune deficiency syndrome (AIDS) results in severe wasting, chronic fatigue, dementia, various opportunistic infections, and certain malignancies (lymphomas and Kaposi's sarcoma) (10). Unless aggressive, combined antire-troviral drug therapy is instituted, the disease is most often fatal. HIV is transmitted by sexual contact, sharing of contaminated needles, transfusion with contaminated blood or transplantation of infected organs, or intrauterine infection of fetuses or transmission through breast milk. HIV-1 is distributed worldwide. HIV-2 infection is similar but milder, usually latent, and rarely progresses to AIDS (12).

Human monkeypox virus. An orthopoxvirus with wide host range, including humans, monkeys, and squirrels, primarily in Africa (22). The clinical appearance of monkeypox in humans is similar to, but less severe than smallpox.

Human papillomaviruses (HPV). HPV are DNA viruses of the papovavirus group that appear to represent at least 100 different viruses. There is some tissue tropism, and several members of the group have strong associations with various cancers. HPV-1 to -4 principally cause skin warts. However, HPV-6 and -11, as well as several higher-numbered members, cause genital warts (condyloma acuminata) that may result in malignant transformation of infected cells. The cancer risk is described as low (HPV-6, -11, -42, -43, and -44), intermediate (HPV-31, -33, -35, -51, and -52), and high (HPV-16, -18, -45, -56, -58, -59, and -68) (42). At least 98% of cervical cancers are caused by various HPV types. In addition, non-melanoma squamous-cell skin cancers are highly associated with HPV, especially types 5 and 8 (13).

HPV are spread via direct contact (touching or sexual contact).

Human polyomaviruses. DNA viruses of the papovavirus group, including BK and JC viruses.

Human T-cell lymphotropic viruses (HTLV). Retroviruses of the oncovirus group.

HTLV-1. Causes adult T-cell leukemia/lymphoma (ATL) that is associated with generalized lymphadenopathy, hepatosplenomegaly, and cutaneous nodular lesions. Complications arise frequently due to impaired immunity and include various opportunistic infections. A second disease caused by HTLV-1 is myelopathy/tropical spastic paraparesis (HAM/TSP) that causes muscle weakness in the legs, hyperflexia, sensory disturbances, and several other severe neurologic symptoms (30). The virus is transmitted by blood and various body fluids similar to the transmission of HIV.

HTLV-2. Causes a neurologic disease similar to HAM/TSP, but is even less common than HTLV-1 infection. It is transmitted in the same manner as HIV and HTLV-1. Screening of the blood supply for both agents is now performed routinely in many countries, including the United States.

Influenza. A group of orthomyxoviruses that can be distinguished as follows:

Influenza A. An endemic or epidemic cause of the "flu" worldwide. Influenza A may cause slightly more severe symptoms of fever, chills, headache, cough, myalgia, and occasionally pneumonia than influenza B or C strains (36). Reye syndrome may occur in children given aspirin during a bout of influenza. Individuals at risk of complications (e.g., bacterial pneumonia) arising from influenza may be vaccinated annually with updated vaccines against influenza A and B. Influenza A viruses are subcategorized based on the major membrane glycoproteins, hemagglutinins, and neuraminidase. It is against these epitopes that influenza vaccines are developed and frequently updated. Influenza A viruses can be transmitted between species, including birds and pigs in addition to humans.

Influenza B. Also an endemic or epidemic cause of the "flu" worldwide. Like influenza A, symptoms include fever, chills, headache, cough, myalgia, and occasionally pneumonia. Reye syndrome may occur in children given aspirin during treatment for influenza.

Influenza C. Much milder and less common than influenza A or B. It may infect pigs as well as humans.

Japanese encephalitis. A mosquito-borne flavivirus that causes asymptomatic to severe disease. It occurs primarily in Asia and India.

JC virus. Causes progressive multifocal leukoencephalopathy (PML), a demyelinating disease of immunocompromised patients (e.g., patients with AIDS, organ transplant recipients) that often proves fatal (33). Many individuals with normal immunity appear to have experienced mild or asymptomatic infection earlier in life. Viral latency may result in reactivation during later periods of cellular immune dysfunction. The virus is thought to be transmitted primarily by respiratory-droplet inhalation, although other routes, including exposure to infected blood or body fluids, cannot be excluded.

Kuru. A fatal neurologic disease found among tribal groups of Papua-New Guinea that is thought to be caused by a prion (25).

Lassa fever. An arenavirus that causes fever, pharyngitis, myalgia, and occasional gastrointestinal bleeding; it can progress to a severe form with multiorgan failure and shock. Lassa fever can be fatal, especially in children, and it can result in fetal loss if infection occurs during pregnancy. It is a zoonotic disease transmitted by aerosols from the urine or feces of rodents in West Africa.

Lentiviruses. Retroviruses including HIV-1 and -2.

Lymphocytic choriomeningitis virus (LCM). An arenavirus that causes predominantly aseptic meningitis with fever, headache, and myalgia (31). It may also cause chorioretinitis, arthritis, myocarditis, and orchitis. It is a zoonotic infection in humans that is contracted by exposure to urine or feces of infected mice in North and South America and Europe.

Lyssavirus. See Rabies.

Marburg virus. See Filoviruses.

Measles. See Rubeola.

Metapneumovirus. Human metapneumovirus (hMPV) is a newly recognized human respiratory virus related to respiratory syncytial virus (RSV) and to avian metapneumovirus. Human metapneumovirus either alone, or as a coinfection with RSV, has caused bronchiolitis in young children. hMPV was initially thought to be involved with severe acute respiratory syndrome (SARS) prior to the discovery of the unique coronavirus SARS agent.

Molluscum contagiosum virus. A cause of small skin tumors of children or genital warts associated with sexual contact in adults. Large skin tumors or disseminated infection can occur in immunocompromised individuals. Lesions tend to spread by auto-inoculation.

Monkeypox virus. An orthopoxvirus first reported in Asian cynomolgus monkeys. It, however, is principally a disease of squirrels, porcupines, and rodents in West and Central Africa. Humans (and probably primates) develop the disease as a zoonosis from direct contact with infected indigenous rodent hosts. The resulting disease in humans strongly resembles smallpox with vesicular and pustular lesions, except that lymphadenopathy is more likely with monkeypox. Persons who have received smallpox vaccine appear to be protected from infection with monkeypox. The first cases in the United States occurred in 2003 when pet prairie dogs infected by a giant Gambian rat transmitted monkeypox to owners and caretakers of the prairie dogs.

Mumps virus. An RNA virus that causes mumps, characterized by fever, fatigue, parotitis, orchitis (adult males), and occasionally aseptic meningitis. It is transmitted by respiratory droplets, but is now largely prevented by vaccination programs in developed countries with MMR (measles-mumps-rubella) vaccine (8).

Noroviruses. Previously called Norwalk-like viruses (NLV). These caliciviruses are the most common cause of gastrointestinal infections in the United States, often in outbreak settings in long-term care facilities, large public gatherings involving food and beverages, and aboard cruise ships. Indeed, many of the outbreaks attributed specifically to Norwalk virus were likely norovirus disease. Many outbreaks, in fact, involved non-food-borne modes of transmission through contaminated surfaces. Noroviruses are particularly stable in the environment and require aggressive disinfection practices to bring outbreaks under control.

Norwalk virus. A calicivirus that causes predominantly gastrointestinal infection in winter months. Norwalk viruses have been associated especially with water-borne outbreaks in communities and aboard cruise ships (24).

Oncoviruses. Retroviruses including HTLV-1 and -2.

Orthomyxoviruses. A group of RNA viruses that include influenza A, B, and C viruses.

Orthopoxvirus. See Poxviruses.

Papovavirus. A small group of DNA viruses that includes human papillomaviruses (HPV) and polyomaviruses.

Parainfluenza virus. A group of four paramyxoviruses (RNA) that cause upper respiratory tract infections. PIV-1 is the principal cause of croup in children, while PIV-2 and PIV-3 also cause croup. PIV-3 is a common cause of bronchiolitis and pneumonia in infants. PIV-4 usually causes mild upper respiratory tract diseases, including the common cold, otitis, and pharyngitis. Transmission is by respiratory droplets, especially among young children.

Paramyxovirus. See Mumps virus and Parainfluenza virus.

Parapoxvirus. Viruses of various animals, including cattle, sheep, and goats. Often causes contagious ecthyma and stomatitis in those animal species, and can cause infections of the hands through contact with infected animals. In a similar manner, humans can acquire milker's nodule from infected dairy cattle.

Parvovirus. The only single-strand DNA viruses, especially including the B-19 virus, a cause of several important diseases. These include erythema infectiosum, a red facial rash ("slapped cheek," also called fifth disease) in children. B-19 infection results in arthritis with or without rash in 50 to 80% of adults, resulting in chronic joint pain in some patients. Perhaps most important is lysis of erythroid precursor cells that can give rise to a fatal aplastic anemia in patients with sickle cell anemia, or chronic anemia in immunosuppressed patients (6). Abortion can result if a mother becomes infected with B-19 during pregnancy. Less important are adeno- and herpes-dependent parvoviruses that may cause coinfections, e.g., dependoviruses.

Picornaviruses. A group of RNA viruses that includes the following:

> **Enteroviruses.** Coxsackie A and B viruses; echoviruses; enteroviruses, especially 70 and 71; hepatitis A virus; polioviruses.

> **Rhinoviruses.** Types 1 to 100+. Large group of respiratory viruses that represent frequent causes of the common cold.

Pneumovirus. See Respiratory syncytial virus.

Poliovirus. An enterovirus that can cause aseptic meningitis and, rarely, paralytic poliomyelitis. Paralytic polio is now quite rare due to widespread vaccination. Various types still exist throughout the world and may be acquired by the fecal-oral route.

Polyomaviruses. These include JC and BK viruses. See also Transmissible spongiform encephalopathies.

Poxviruses. The largest and most complex DNA viruses that include especially the orthopoxviruses, vaccinia and variola, monkeypox, cowpox, and the unclassified poxvirus, molluscum contagiosum. All of the poxviruses that infect humans are zoonotic agents, except for molluscum contagiosum and smallpox.

Prions. Proteinaceous infectious particles. Prions differ from true viruses because they are composed of only protein and contain no nucleic acids. Creutzfeldt-Jakob disease (CJD) is a severe, transmissible neurologic syndrome possibly caused by a prion. See also Transmissible spongiform encephalopathies.

Rabies virus. An RNA virus that causes the disease rabies in various animal species, and occasionally humans, in most parts of the world. It causes severe encephalitis manifested as hydrophobia and aerophobia. It is most often fatal, but may be prevented by vaccination of individuals with possible occupational exposures. It is a zoonotic disease transmitted principally by the bite of an infected animal or via body fluids of an infected human (32).

Reoviruses. A group of RNA viruses that includes rotavirus and coltivirus (primarily Colorado tick fever).

Respiratory syncytial virus (RSV). A paramyxovirus that frequently causes upper respiratory tract infections and is the most frequent cause of lower respiratory tract infections in young children. It is highly transmissible by respiratory droplets, especially during the winter months, and often results in local outbreaks of several months' duration (18).

Retroviruses. A group of highly important RNA viruses including the oncoviruses, HTLV-1 and -2, and the lentiviruses, HIV-1 and -2.

Reye syndrome. See Varicella-zoster virus and influenza A and B.

Rhabdovirus. Includes the lyssavirus, rabies.

Rhinoviruses. A large group of picornaviruses (approximately 100 serotypes) that represent the major virus group associated with the common cold. In addition to a self-limited but very uncomfortable cause of rhinorrhea, rhinoviruses can cause sinusitis, otitis, and lower respiratory tract infections. Transmission occurs by respiratory droplets, by hand-to-hand contact, and by contaminated fomites (19).

Rotavirus. Rotaviruses (serogroups A through G) are a group of RNA viruses that cause gastroenteritis in adults and especially in children. Rotavirus A is a very common cause of diarrhea in children, particularly in the winter months (41). Rotaviruses are transmitted by the fecal-oral route.

Rubella. The German measles (3-day measles), caused by a Rubi (Toga) RNA virus. Rubella is characterized by fever and maculopapular rash on the face initially, and then the extremities. In the past, it caused measles epidemics. Today, immunization is commonly performed in developed countries. Congenital rubella can result in serious birth defects involving the eyes, heart, and central nervous system of the fetus (27). It is transmitted by respiratory droplets and by transplacental infection of a fetus. Children in most developed countries are now immunized with the MMR (measles-mumps-rubella) vaccine.

Rubeola. A paramyxovirus that causes measles (7-day measles), characterized by cough, fever, red spots on the oral mucosa (Koplik's spots), and rash on the face, trunk, and eventually the extremities (9). It is highly communicable by respiratory droplets. Children in most developed countries are now immunized with the MMR (measles-mumps-rubella) vaccine.

Rubivirus. See Rubella.

Sapporo-like viruses. A group of caliciviruses that cause diarrhea and vomiting, usually without fever or further symptoms. They occur more frequently in the winter months and are spread by contaminated food or water (4).

SARS. Severe acute respiratory syndrome, a recently described syndrome thought to be due to a unique coronavirus acquired at first in southern China, but which thereafter spread to Hong Kong, Singapore, Vietnam, Canada, and the United States (26, 28).

Smallpox. See Variola virus.

St. Louis encephalitis. A flavivirus transmitted by mosquitoes that can result in severe infection, especially among the elderly. It can be encountered during the warmer months in various areas of the United States.

Thogotovirus. So far, a rare cause of tick-borne disease in some mammals and rarely humans.

Togaviruses. A group of RNA viruses that include a lipid envelope. The group includes alphaviruses and rubiviruses.

Toroviruses. A group of RNA viruses similar to coronaviruses that cause diarrhea in various animals, and probably in humans.

Transmissible spongiform encephalopathies. A group of "slow" virus infections that often progress to a fatal outcome over a long period of time. While the agents are not fully elucidated, some have been described as prions or defective virus particles. The diseases include Creutzfeldt-Jakob disease (CJD), an uncommon, infectious cause of dementia in humans. Kuru was a neurologic disease thought to be transferred through the practice of cannibalism in New Guinea. Of more recent interest, bovine spongiform encephalopathy (BSE or "mad cow disease") is a neurologic disease of cattle that attracted a great deal of media attention in the early 1990s in the United Kingdom because of the fear of its possible spread to humans. Scrapie is a similar disease in sheep and goats in the United Kingdom, Europe, and the United States. While there has been some epidemiologic evidence that BSE might lead to a variety of CJD in humans, no such link has been found with scrapie.

Vaccinia virus. The virus used to prepare the live, attenuated smallpox vaccine. It was historically the cause of cowpox, a condition of the fingers caused by milking infected cows. Now, cowpox, rarely, or a subtype called buffalopox, still exists in a few parts of the world and may infect humans through contact with bovines or other species.

Varicella-zoster virus (VZV). The cause of chicken pox, characterized by progressive stages of skin lesions, which can also result in severe disseminated infections in immunocompromised individuals. Children may develop Reye syndrome from aspirin use during treatment for chicken pox. Adults can have a latent infection called herpes zoster or "shingles" that results from reactivation of latent VZV infection due to stress or immunosuppression. It is manifest as painful vesicular lesions within sensory ganglia of midsection dermatomes, where the viruses maintained latency.

Variola virus. The cause of smallpox, a severe infection characterized by high fever, headache, vomiting, and a severe vesicular rash on the face and trunk that spreads to the extremities. There are two strains or variants: Variola Major associated with a high mortality rate due to spread to internal organs (~ 50% mortality), and Variola Minor that is rarely fatal. Because of intensive public health initiatives, especially vaccination in earlier periods, smallpox has been eliminated globally as a naturally occurring infection (14). However, it remains as a prime candidate for bioterrorism due to waning immunity in most populations. Variola is transmitted by respiratory droplets or by contact with virus from vesicular lesions or scabs.

Venezuelan equine encephalitis. See Alphaviruses.

West Nile virus. A neurotropic arbovirus that may cause mild illness characterized by fever and headache. However, some individuals experience aseptic meningitis and diffuse myelitis. Infection occurs following the bite of an infected mosquito. The natural host of West Nile virus appears to be various species of migrating or local birds.

Western equine encephalitis virus. See Alphaviruses.

Yatapoxviruses. Uncommon members of the paramyxovirus group that cause zoonotic infections from monkeys to humans in Africa, either by direct contact or possibly through biting insects. Infections in humans are generally limited to fever and skin lesions on the extremities or torso.

Yellow fever. A flavivirus that can cause severe infection in humans in South America and Africa. It is transmitted by mosquitoes that have fed on virus-infected monkeys. Mosquito-control efforts have largely eradicated the infection in North and Central America.

SUGGESTED READINGS

1. Bennet, J. V., and P. S. Brachman (ed.). 1998. *Hospital Infections*, 4th ed. Lippincott-Raven, Philadelphia, Pa.

2. Forbes, B. A., D. F. Sahm, and A. S. Weisfeld (ed.). 2002. *Bailey and Scott's Diagnostic Microbiology*, 11th ed. Mosby-Year Book, St. Louis, Mo.

3. Gilbert, D. N., R. C. Moellering, Jr., and M. A. Sande. 2003. *The Sanford Guide to Antimicrobial Therapy*, 33rd ed. Antimicrobial Therapy, Inc., Hyde Park, Vt.

4. Gorbach, S. L., J. G. Bartlett, and N. R. Blacklow (ed.). 1997. *Infectious Diseases*, 2nd ed. W.B. Saunders, Philadelphia, Pa.

5. Jenson, H. B., and R. S. Baltimore. 2002. *Pediatric Infectious Diseases: Principles and Practices*. The W. B. Saunders Co., Philadelphia, Pa.

6. Knipe, D. M., P. M. Howley, D. E. Griffin, R. A. Lamb, M. A. Martin, B. Roizman, and S. E. Straus (ed.). 2001. *Fields Virology*, 4th ed. Lipincott, Williams & Wilkins, Philadelphia, Pa.

7. Koneman, E. W., S. D. Allen, W. J. Janda, P. C. Schreckenberger, and W. C. Winn, Jr., (ed.). 1997. *Color Atlas and Textbook of Diagnostic Microbiology*, 5th ed. Lippincott, Philadelphia, Pa.

8. Mahy, B. W. J., and L. Collier (ed.). 1998. *Topley and Wilson's Microbiology and Microbial Infections*, vol. 1. Arnold, London, United Kingdom.

9. Mandell, G. L., J. E. Bennett, and R. Dolin (ed.). 2000. *Mandell, Douglas and Bennett's Principles and Practice of*

Infectious Diseases, 5th ed. Churchill Livingstone, New York, N.Y.

10. Murray, P. R., E. J. Baron, J. H. Jorgensen, M. A. Pfaller, and R. H. Yolken (ed.). 2003. *Manual of Clinical Microbiology*, 8th ed. ASM Press, Washington, D.C.

11. Murray, P. R., K. S. Rosenthal, G. S. Kobayashi, and M. A. Pfaller (ed.). 2002. *Medical Microbiology*, 4th ed. Mosby-Year Book, St. Louis, Mo.

12. Schaechter, M., C. Engleberg, B. I. Eisenstein, and G. Medoff (ed.). 1999. *Mechanisms of Microbial Diseases*, 3rd ed. Williams & Wilkins, Baltimore, Md.

13. Specter, S., R. L. Hodinka, and S. A. Yount. 2000. *Clinical Virology Manual*, 3rd ed. ASM Press, Washington, D.C.

REFERENCES

1. **Alter, M. J.** 1997. Epidemiology of hepatitis C. *Hepatology* **26**(3 Suppl. 1):62S–65S.

2. **Alter, H. J., Y. Nakatsuji, J. Melpolder, J. Wages, R. Wesley, J. W. Shih, and J. P. Kim.** 1997. The incidence of hepatitis G virus infection and its relation to liver disease. *N. Engl. J. Med.* **336**:747–754.

3. **Arthur, R., K. Shah, S. Baust, G. Santos, and R. Saral.** 1986. Association of BK viruria with hemorrhagic cystis in recipients of bone marrow transplants. *N. Engl. J. Med.* **315**:230–234.

4. **Blacklow, N. R., and H. B. Greenberg.** 1991. Viral gastroenteritis. *N. Engl. J. Med.* **325**:252–264.

5. **Braun, D. K., G. Dominguez, and P. E. Pellett.** 1997. Human herpesvirus 6. *Clin. Microbiol. Rev.* **10**:521–567.

6. **Brown, K. E., and N. S. Young.** 1995. Parvovirus B19 infection and hematopoiesis. *Blood Rev.* **9**:176–182.

7. **Centers for Disease Control and Prevention.** 1998. Fatal cercopithevcine herpesvirus 1 (B virus) infection following mucocutaneous exposure and interim recommendations for worker protection. *Morb. Mortal. Wkly. Rep.* **47**:1073–1076.

8. **Centers for Disease Control and Prevention.** 1998. Measels, mumps, and rubella-vaccine use and strategies for elimination of measles, rubella, and congenital rubella syndrome and control of mumps: recommendations of the Advisory Committee on Immunization Practices (ACIP). *Morb. Mortal. Wkly. Rep.* **47**(RR-8):6–16.

9. **Centers for Disease Control and Prevention.** 2002. Measles—United States, 2000. *Morb. Mortal. Wkly. Rep.* **51**:120–123.

10. **Centers for Disease Control and Prevention.** 1992. 1993 revised classification system for HIV infection and expanded surveillance case definition for AIDS among adolescents and adults. *Morb. Mortal. Wkly. Rep.* **41**:1–19.

11. **Chang, Y., E. Caesarman, M. S. Pessin, F. Lee, J. Culpepper, D. M. Knowles, and P. S. Moore.** 1994. Identification of herpesvirus-like DNA sequences in AIDS-associated Kaposi's sarcoma. *Science* **266**:1865–1869.

12. **Clavel, F., M. Guyander, D. Gustaard, M. Salle, L. Montagnier, and M. Alizon.** 1986. Molecular cloning

and polymorphism of the human immune deficiency virus type 2. *Nature* **324**:691–695.

13. de Villiers, E. M., A. Ruhland, and P. Sekaric. 1999. Human papillomaviruses in nonmelanoma skin cancer. *Semin. Cancer Biol.* **9**:413–422.

14. Fenner, F., D. A. Henderson, I. Arita, Z. Jezek, and I. Ladnyi. 1988. *Smallpox and Its Eradication*. World Health Organization, Geneva, Switzerland.

15. Fleming, D. T., G. McQuillan, R. E., Johnson, A. J. Nahmias, S. O. Aral, F. K. Lee, and M. E. St. Louis. 1997. Herpes simplex virus type 2 in the United States, 1976 to 1994. *N. Engl. J. Med.* **337**:1105–1111.

16. Ghani, A. C., C. A. Donelly, N. M. Ferguson, and R. M. Anderson. 2002. The transmission dynamics of BSE and vCJD. *C. R. Acad Sci. Ser. III* **325**:37–47.

17. Gibbons, R. V., R. C. Holman, E. D. Belay, and L. B. Schonberger. 2000. Creutzfeldt-Jakob disease in the United States: 1979–1998. *JAMA* **284**:2322–2323.

18. Hall, C. B. 1999. Respiratory syncytial virus: a continuing culprit and conundrum. *J. Pediatr.* **135**:2–7.

19. Hendley, J. O. 1999. Clinical virology of rhinoviruses. *Adv. Virus Res.* **54**:453–466.

20. Hermann, J. E., D. N. Taylor, P. Echeverria, and N. R. Blacklow. 1991. Astrovirus as a cause of gastroenteritis in children. *N. Engl. J. Med.* **324**:1757–1760.

21. Hsu, J. L., and S. L. Glaser. 2000. Epstein-Barr virus-associated malignancies: epidemiologic patterns and etiologic implications. *Crit. Rev. Oncol. Hematol.* **34**:27–53.

22. **Hutin, Y. J. F., R. J. Williams, P. Malfait, R. Pebody, V. N. Loparev, S. L. Ropp, M. Rodriguez, J. C. Knight, F. K. Tschioko, A. S. Khan, M. V. Szczeniowaki, and J. J. Esposito.** 2001. Outbreak of human monkeypox, Democratic Republic of Congo. *Emerg. Infect. Dis.* 7: 434–438.

23. **Jahrling, P. B., T. W. Geisbert, J. B. Geisbert, J. R. Swearengen, M. Bray, N. K. Jaax, J. W. Huggins, J. W. LeDuc, and C. J. Peters.** 1990. Preliminary report: isolation of Ebola virus from monkeys imported to the USA. *Lancet* 335:502–505.

24. **Kaplan, J. E., G. W. Gary, R. C. Baron, N. Singh, L. B. Schonberger, R. Feldman, and H. B. Greenberg.** 1982. Epidemiology of Norwalk gastroenteritis and the role of Norwalk virus in outbreaks of acute nonbacterial gastroenteritis. *Ann. Intern. Med.* 96:756–761.

25. **Klitzman, R. L., M. P. Alpers, and D. C. Gajdusek.** 1984. The natural incubation period of kuru and the episodes of transmission in three clusters of patients. *Neuroepidemiology* 3:3–20.

26. **Ksiazek, T. G., D. Erdman, C. S. Goldsmith, S. R. Zaki, T. Peret, S. Emery, S. Tong, C. Urbani, J. A. Comer, W. Lim, P. E. Rollin, S. F. Dowell, A.-E. Ling, C. D. Humphrey, W.-J. Shieh, J. Guarner, C. D. Paddock, P. Rota, B. Fields, J. DeRisi, J.-Y. Yang, N. Cox, J. M. Hughes, J. W. LeDuc, W. J. Bellini, and L. J. Anderson.** 2003. A novel coronavirus associated with severe acute respiratory syndrome. *N. Engl. J. Med.* 348:1953–1966.

27. **Lee, J.-Y., and D. S. Bowden.** 2000. Rubella virus replication and links to teratogenicity. *Clin. Microbiol. Rev.* **13**:571–587.

28. **Lee, N., D. Hui, A. Wu, P. Chan, P. Cameron, G. M. Joynt, A. Ahuja, M. Y. Yung, C. B. Leung, K. F. To, S. F. Lui, C. C. Szeto, S. Chung, and J. J. Y. Sung.** 2003. A major outbreak of severe acute respiratory syndrome in Hong Kong. *N. Engl. J. Med.* **348**:1986–1994.

29. **Mahoney, F. J.** 1999. Update on diagnosis, management, and prevention of hepatitis B virus infection. *Clin. Microbiol. Rev.* **12**:351–366.

30. **Manns, A., M. Hisada, and L. La Grange.** 1999. Human T-lymphotropic virus type 1 infection. *Lancet* **353**:1951–1958.

31. **Mets, M. B., L. J. Barton, A. S. Khan, and T. G. Ksiazek.** 2000. Lymphocytic choriomeningitis virus: an underdiagnosed cause of congenital chorioretinitis. *Am. J. Ophthalmol.* **130**:209–215.

32. **Noah, D. L., C. L. Drenzek, J. S. Smith, J. W. Krebs, L. A. Orcaiari, J. Shaddock, D. Sanderlin, S. Whitfield, M. Fekadu, J. G. Olson, C. E. Ruprecht, and J. E. Childs.** 1998. Epidemiology of human rabies in the United States, 1980–1996. *Ann. Intern. Med.* **128**:922–930.

33. **Padget, B. L., C. M. Rogers, and D. L. Walker.** 1977. JC virus, a human polyomavirus associated with progressive multifocal leukoencephalopathy: additional biological characteristics and antigenic relationships. *Infect. Immun.* **15**:656–662.

34. Pichichero, M. F., S. McLinn, H. A. Rotbart, M. A. Menegus, M. Casciano, and B. E. Reidenberg. 1998. Clinical and economic impact of enterovirus illness in private pediatric practice. *Pediatrics* **102**:1126–1134.

35. Schmaljohn, C., and B. Hjelle. 1997. Hantaviruses: a global problem. *Emerg. Infect. Dis.* **3**:95–104.

36. Simonsen, L., K. Fukuda, L. B. Shonberger, and N. J. Cox. 2000. The impact of influenza epidemics on hospitalizations. *J. Infect. Dis.* **181**:831–837.

37. Smedile, A., M. Rizzetto, and J. L. Gerin. 1994. Advances in hepatitis D virus biology and disease. *Prog. Liver Dis.* **12**:157–175.

38. Smith, J. L. 2001. A review of hepatitis E virus. *J. Food Prot.* **64**:572–586.

39. Spruance, S. L. 1992. The natural history of recurrent oral-facial herpes simplex virus infection. *Semin. Dermatol.* **11**:200–206.

40. Strader, D. B., and L. B. Seeff. 1996. New hepatitis A vaccines and their role in prevention. *Drugs* **51**:359–366.

41. Waters, V., E. L. Ford-Jones, M. Petric, M. Fearon, P. Corey, R. Moineddein, and the Pediatric Rotavirus Epidemiology Study for Immunization Study Group. 2000. Etiology of community-acquired pediatric viral diarrhea: a prospective longitudinal study in hospitals, emergency departments, pediatric practices and child care centers during the winter rotavirus outbreak, 1997–1998. *Pediatr. Infect. Dis. J.* **19**:843–848.

42. Xi, L. F., L. A. Koutsky, D. A. Galloway, J. Kuypers, J. P. Hughes, C. M. Wheeler, K. K. Holmes, and N. B.

Kiviat. 1997. Genomic variation of human papillomaviruses type 16 and risk for high grade cervical intraepithelial neoplasia. *J. Natl. Cancer Inst.* 89:796–802.